# MEDICAL SCHOOL ADMISSIONS:
## The Insider's Guide

*3rd Revised Edition*

**John A. Zebala**

**Daniel B. Jones**

**Stephanie B. Jones**

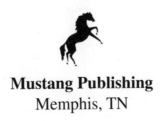

**Mustang Publishing**
Memphis, TN

Distributed to the trade in the USA by National Book Network, Lanham, Maryland.

**Library of Congress Cataloging in Publication Data**
Zebala, John A., 1965-
    Medical school admissions : the insider's guide / John
A. Zebala, Daniel B. Jones, Stephanie B. Jones. -- 3rd
revised ed.
        p.   cm.
    ISBN 0-914457-71-3
    1. Medical colleges--United States--Admissions.
2. Medical colleges--United States--Entrance requirements.
I. Jones, Daniel B., 1964-   . II. Jones, Stephanie B.
(Stephanie Brickner) III. Title.
R838.4.Z42   1994
610' .71'173--dc20                                        94-32790
                                                          CIP

Printed on acid-free paper.

10 9 8 7 6 5 4 3

Wherever the art
of medicine is loved,
there is also love
of humanity.

—Hippocrates

# Acknowledgments

This book is dedicated to Keith Bernstein, Doug Lytle, Steve Taylor, Brian Wong, Francis Barany, Mary Burton, Carol Snow, Alfonso Torres, Jane Crawford, and Amy Burnham—undergraduate and graduate friends without whose knowledge, inspiration, and sometimes irritation this book would have never been written.

We would also like to thank the many Deans of Admission who gave thoughtful commentary on this book.

Special thanks also to the students accepted at Cornell University Medical College, Johns Hopkins, Yale, Harvard, UCLA, University of Pennsylvania, Columbia, Washington University, and New York University who contributed their successful essays. These students include (but are not limited to) Wendell Danforth, John Linsalata, Matt Pease, Jeff Budoff, Hal Baker, Dan Medalie, Karl Illig, Daniel Javit, Fred Lee, Perry Sutaria, and Marcia Simpson.

Thanks to Greg Sicard, Jr. for his input during the preparation of the third edition.

Most important, we would like to thank our parents, who supported us throughout the admissions process not too long ago.

*John A. Zebala*
*Daniel B. Jones*
*Stephanie B. Jones*

# Foreword

At present, over 40,000 individuals apply for the 16,000 positions available yearly at the medical schools in the United States. Both applicants and schools take the annual application process most seriously and expend a great deal of time and effort making it work favorably for them.

To insure consistency and continuity, most medical school admissions committee members serve more than one annual processing cycle. In contrast, students attempt to navigate the course from applicant to matriculant only once. Therefore, it's most reasonable for them to ask at the beginning, "What can I do to help my chances of being selected by the school of my choice?"

In what follows, John Zebala, Daniel Jones, and Stephanie Jones—successful applicants to medical schools—offer their firsthand account of "what works." For those who endured the admissions process several decades ago, it is an eyeopening account of the present. For those seeking to start the path towards a medical education, it is a thought-provoking collection of organized steps and considerations for your assistance.

In practice, the medical school admissions process initially reduces you, the individual, to several sets of numbers (GPAs and MCAT scores), lists of courses and accomplishments, an essay, and several letters of recommendation. In short, it makes you create a paper caricature of yourself. Next, admissions committees review thousands of such "paper individuals" to select a group of manageable size to interview. Finally, from the hundreds interviewed, a few individuals are admitted to fill classes of 90 to 170.

How do you survive this process and effectively represent

yourself? The authors offer their thoughts on doing just that. Is everything they suggest suitable for every applicant? Of course not. But you should consider their suggestions and decide which are suitable for you. It's certainly helpful and worth your time.

Remember, medical school admissions committees are seeking intelligent, thoughtful, caring, motivated individuals to fill their classes. To be successful, you must demonstrate those qualities that suit you for entering the medical profession, as well as those that make you a unique, interesting individual.

My advice: Be yourself, and don't let the real you get lost in the process.

Gordon F. Fairclough, Jr., Ph.D.
*Dean of Admissions*
*Cornell University Medical College*

# Contents

# Introduction

One of the most difficult things to do when applying to medical school is to decipher which advice is accurate and which is not. The main problem is that most of the people giving advice have never actually gone through the admissions process themselves. That's why this book is unique.

As recent medical students, we have firsthand knowledge of the admissions process that will probably be the best and most realistic advice you'll ever hear. Often, books and counselors do more to *dis*courage the applicant than *en*courage. Well, we're not going to tell you that in order to be a doctor you have to make straight A's, climb Mount Everest, or be Ms. Wonderful-Everything, because the fact is you don't.

We believe that getting into medical school is not an insurmountable task, and that what most doctors actually do in their everyday practice does not require a genius intellect or qualify them for a Nobel Prize. Instead, we believe that the whole admissions process is a formula, a game with set rules. If you play the game by the rules, you'll get in. It's that simple. Our goal is to tell you exactly what the formula entails, as we have learned from our own experience and from interviews with admissions committee members.

**The best effect of any book is that it excites the reader to self activity.**
*—Thomas Carlyle*

A major attraction in our book, we believe, is the large number of actual application essays (a.k.a. "personal statements") collected from students admitted to top medical colleges around the country. Applicants can spend months writing and perfecting their essays, and every year premedical students scramble and search for successful essays to read. We think the collection will be invaluable in showing you how broad the range of potential topics is, and it should give you an idea of what gets admissions committees excited. Plus, we hope the essays will inspire your own creativity and relieve some anxiety.

Another extremely anxious time for the applicant to medical school is the interview. The uncertainties and fears surrounding this part of the process can be a nightmare. So, we have accumulated a list of questions that interviewers have asked applicants during actual interviews. We have also researched what interviewers typically seek during an interview. Applicants rarely know how their application and responses are evaluated, or what questions are likely to arise in the interview. These pieces of information are exactly what you need to turn what might be just good interviews into really great interviews.

We also recommend additional reading, rank the country's medical schools, provide the latest information on the MCAT, and include a timetable that allows you to track and check your progress throughout the application process.

Most important, we encourage premedical students to apply with confidence, and we suggest ways they can properly market their strengths.

It may also be useful to mention what this book is *not*. This book will not help you decide if medicine is the right career for you. That decision can come only from working in a hospital and observing physicians. Also, we make no attempt to glorify medicine; we'll leave that to *General Hospital* and *M\*A\*S\*H*. Instead, we hope to convince you that half the battle in the medical school admissions game is thinking positively and knowing how to work within the system.

Once you have these insights, you'll realize that it's not necessary to be cutthroat to get into medical school. On the contrary, the best physicians are not chemistry lab nerds who would sabotage a neighbor's experiment. They are thoughtful, caring, well-rounded people with wide-ranging interests. If you would like to be this kind of physician, read on, because what follows is the ultimate set of insider's tips for medical school admissions success!

# Chapter 1

# Premedical Preparation

B asically, there are three types of premedical students. The first is the most familiar. They knew they were going to be physicians from the very beginning. At age two, they were playing with stethoscopes. In high school, they chose a college based on how it would affect their medical school acceptance. The second and probably largest group are those who decided to undertake the quest for medical school in their undergraduate years. The third group consists of people who decided on med school after college graduation—and sometimes after being established in another career.

While different in many ways, all three groups share two common misconceptions. First, they think that just because medicine draws upon science, every premed should major in biology or chemistry. Second, they think the quality of their college and their major are decisive factors in their admission to medical school.

In fact, nothing could be further from the truth. Because the spectrum of physicians is so broad, there is no preferred major to enter the medical profession. In some cases, the quality of the undergraduate university can affect your chances of admission to medical school, but usually it's irrelevant. (An important exception are undergraduate colleges that have an affiliated medical school. More on this later.)

Despite worries over physicians' incomes shrinking because of health care reform measures, the March 1994 issue of *Money Magazine* ranks "physician" as the second-best job in America, after "computer systems analyst" (and who wants to do that?). So it's not too surprising that many premedical student are conscious (almost paranoid) about the most minor details of their undergraduate curriculum. The unfortunate reality is that the paranoia is unfounded. It's based on pervasive myths spread by other premedical students, not on the true details that admissions committees consider important.

So what *is* important? At the risk of over-simplifying, you must have (or create) a quality that makes you stand out from the pack. Standing out is another way of saying that you are "interesting," and "interesting" is what medical schools go for.

Once you decide to pursue medical school, it's essential that you remain you. It's okay to explore your talents and curiosity in college (indeed, we heartily recommend it). Go ahead and learn to scuba dive or take a course on Emily Dickinson, if that's what you'd like to do. With this philosophy, you need not worry about the person next to you all the time, and you'll be much more relaxed. If you want to become a "doctor to the stars" in Hollywood, get a degree in business or, better yet, film. Don't laugh! Patients want to be able to relate to their doctors.

If you are like most premedical students, you probably don't know what kind of doctor you want to become. So our advice is simple: major in whatever interests you.

## Planning Your Undergraduate Study

When medical schools receive an applicant's grades, they look at the overall grade point average, as well as the GPA derived exclusively from science courses.

Now, you non-science majors probably realize your potential disadvantage in this procedure. That is, if an English major gets a C in freshman chemistry, he'll have a pitiful science grade point average, because he won't have many science courses to average with the C. That lone C will stand as indicative of mediocre scientific ability—though it may in

> **In the long run of history, the censor and the inquisitor have always lost. The only sure weapon against bad ideas is better ideas. The source of better ideas is wisdom. The surest path to wisdom is a liberal education.**
>
> —*A. Whitney Griswold*

fact be a false representation.

We know all the sob stories about your bad semester that year. You had family problems, girl- or boyfriend problems, a lingering case of beriberi, etc. Unfortunately, while these stories are often true and relevant, medical schools give little if any consideration to such deficiencies unless you show marked improvement and progress later in your transcript.

So if you're a non-science major and you've got a poor science grade, you'll need to spend extra effort to raise your science average. If your grade is poor in a course, take the course again if you can get the bad grade erased. If you can't get it erased but merely averaged with the new grade, we don't advise taking the course over. Instead, take a more advanced science course, which will average the low grade plus look better and more purposeful on your transcript.

Medical schools today seem to have had enough of the eggheads, and they are leaning more towards people with degrees in the liberal arts and science majors who are "well-rounded." In fact, economics majors have some of the highest percentages of acceptance to medical colleges, and biology majors among the lowest, within each of their respective groups. (Of course, this doesn't mean you should switch your major to economics, because an alternative interpretation of this statistic is possible. That is, a higher percentage of mediocre applicants are biology majors, since nearly every biology major applies to med school.)

We have a friend, a straight-A biomedical engineer, who interviewed at Washington University. One of the first things they told him was, "Frankly, Mr. Smith, we've found that English majors make the best doctors." Don't get us wrong—he had no trouble getting accepted there. The point is, it's wrong to think that you must be a science major to be a doctor, or that being a science major will give you an advantage when applying to medical school.

A premedical student must fulfill certain science requirements: one year of inorganic chemistry, one year of organic chemistry, one year of physics, and one year of biology. Other required subjects, such as English and calculus, vary with different med schools. Past these, you can study almost anything you want.

At many schools, the science courses are extremely difficult, especially at schools with a good science reputation. This is also often the case at large universities, where classes with over 700 premedical students are common. Usually, organic chemistry is the "weed-out" class. Well, here's some good news: you don't need to be part of a "weed-out," and you don't have to sit back and take it. If you can take organic elsewhere, where it's easier and maybe even cheaper, then by all means do so. An A is an A on your transcript, no matter where you got it. However, make certain your college will allow you to transfer the course credit before you spend your summer in a classroom.

All of you have heard people say that they were going to take so-and-so science course because they thought it would help them in medical school or look good to admissions committees. This is the most absurd way of assuring yourself an A or an honors later in medical school. Med schools apparently agree with us, since most discourage students from taking courses that resemble the first year's curriculum. (Genetics and biochemistry are occasional exceptions.)

The best way to get an A in med school is simply to work hard for it when the time comes. Unless you are truly interested in the sciences, you will not make your transcript look more impressive by taking med school-level courses as an undergraduate. In fact, you'll probably make it look worse, because your grade point average will be lower. Anyway, when you don't have to worry about advanced courses, you'll have more time to go to the beach or the mountains.

The hardest hurdle to jump is getting into a medical

school. Therefore, any method that lets you take short cuts, have fun, and still get in is a perfectly acceptable alternative to killing yourself by studying 24 hours a day for courses that you may never use again in your life.

The rationale is simple: you'll learn everything you need to know to become a doctor in medical school. You don't need to be Isaac Newton's clone, and you don't need advanced courses on the undergraduate level. You simply must show aptitude and a minimum amount of knowledge about science so you can survive the medical curriculum.

Completing your undergraduate degree with good grades merely tells a medical college you have the *stamina* to persevere for four years, and do it well. In general, it's a good indication of your ability to do well in medical school, because the coursework in med school is just like undergraduate coursework, but at much higher endurance levels.

## Picking the Right Undergraduate College

Many medical schools will tell applicants from junior colleges and some state universities that, statistically, they are at a distinct disadvantage to applicants who went to a private university or a respected state school. The reason is that GPAs earned at the former are not deemed as valuable as those from more competitive schools. We agree that this is unfair, especially since many people must attend such schools for economic or geographic reasons.

So what do you do if you go to Mediocre State Tech? Pack it up and transfer? Certainly not! You'll just have to be that much better than the others, and your GPA should be that much higher.

**It is all one to me if a man comes from Sing Sing or Harvard. We hire a man, not his history. —Henry Ford**

Does this mean that med schools make numerical adjustments on GPAs depending on what college you attended? Yes, many do. Obviously, this hurts individuals high on the scale whose grades are adjusted down, since it's impossible to achieve higher than a 4.0 average. On the other hand, admissions committees often inflate the value of grades from prestigious colleges, so a lot of boneheads get in from top schools. Hey, who said life is fair?

You basically have two choices: transfer to a better school, if that's the problem, or work really hard where you are. We favor doing the latter, rather than worrying about the alma mater.

However, there is one case when we suggest you transfer. If you have the choice, always go to a university with a medical school. Twenty percent of the students at some medical schools attended that school as an undergraduate. Obviously, the university must show that it believes in its own product, so, statistically, its own premeds have a notable advantage over other applicants when they apply to their university's med school.

Nevertheless, if you are good, it doesn't matter where you went to college. You'll stand out sooner or later. Besides, medical colleges have devised a way out of such subjective dilemmas—it's called the MCAT. It turns all students—whether they're from Yale or Arkansas Tech—into an objective number. If you do well on the MCAT, you'll likely get into medical school.

So don't lose sleep about which undergraduate school you should attend. Go to the college that appeals to you because of location, price, curriculum, sports program, or other personal reasons. If chemistry and physics are your thing, then go to a school known for sciences. The same logic applies if you're interested in drama or art.

The real bottom line is how you measure up as a person. College may give you the only opportunity to enjoy and explore things that really excite you other than medicine. After all, health professionals treat people and must be personable, not simply mechanics fixing machines. They must have a well-rounded intelligence, as well as scientific knowledge, since they deal with incredible technology—and everyday patients.

So don't be one-dimensional, the stereotypical premed nerd, grinding away for hours in the library and the lab. Use your undergraduate experience creatively and explore college opportunities to their fullest. It will do wonders to shape you as a whole person, and it will make you a much better doctor someday.

## *Post-Baccalaureate Programs*

Designed to get people into medical school after they have already graduated from college, post-baccalaureate programs are especially attractive to older applicants who have decided midway through a different career to pursue medicine but lack the necessary premed course requirements. Dr. W. Edwin Dodson, Dean of Admissions at Washington University in St. Louis, sees such programs springing up all over the place. As to whether they help, "outcome is directly related to cause," he said. Students who fall back on post-baccalaureate programs to remedy a poor undergraduate performance are less likely to benefit than engineers who simply lack a few required courses. Each program's record must also be taken into account. The University of Pennsylvania and Columbia University, for example, both have high placement records and are surely doing something right. Other schools' records are spotty, so *caveat emptor*.

There are too many post-baccalaureate programs for us to list here. For more information, call the medical schools you're interested in attending. Their admissions offices should be able to point you in the right direction.

# Chapter 2

# Power Techniques for Higher Grades

I t's common knowledge that good grades are essential for gaining acceptance to medical school. The problem is, "good" is rarely defined.

For those who don't have perfect grade point averages, the belief that "the higher the GPA, the better" can cause some real mental anguish — especially if you use the class valedictorian as your standard. On the other hand, you're kidding yourself if you think medical schools admit students at the bottom of their class. Of course, reality is somewhere between these two extremes.

Here's a real life example: During our volunteer work in an urban emergency room, a physician told us he had a 2.0 average as an undergraduate majoring in chemistry. After graduation, he didn't know what he wanted to do with his life, so he went to Africa with the Peace Corps for two years. Helping a lot of suffering people there convinced him that medicine was his calling. He returned to the United States and took a year of graduate courses, after which he entered medical school.

In contrast, we know an applicant from a prestigious college who had nearly perfect grades and MCAT scores. Almost every medical school rejected him. The problem was that nothing in his record made him unique or revealed a sincere desire to study medicine.

The lesson, then, is simple: there's not always a clear grade break determining who will and who won't be accepted. In fact, some medical schools don't even have a minimum GPA requirement. For the sake of being realistic though, you should have at least a 3.0—unless your MCAT scores are quite high or you have special circumstances in your personal life.

Some of you may think such grades are difficult to attain. However, we believe a 3.0 or higher is a realistic goal for just about anybody, if you go about it correctly.

## *Techniques for Grade Point Success*

Although you may be familiar with some of the techniques outlined in this chapter, many people do not adhere to even the most basic points. The irony is, those who don't practice good study habits are often the same students who complain about how difficult their courses are. Therefore, if you fall into this group, or even if you don't, refresh your memory about good, basic study techniques. These concepts can make your courses seem much easier.

**1. Obtain old exams.** The first golden rule to success in college courses is to study old exams. Professors are not so creative that they can devise original exam questions each year. In fact, they often don't have time to change the test much at all. So you'll frequently see either the same or very similar questions on old exams.

Some of you may think, "I don't need old exams, because if I really know the material I'll ace the exam anyway." We thought the same thing until reality (and a few C's) hit us in the face. Many questions that involve concepts require insight from the student, and insight requires time—usually more time than allowed on exams. Exposure to similar or identical concepts days before an exam will put you way ahead of others who are seeing the problem for the first time.

Using this technique, a two-letter increase in your grades is common (i.e., from a C to an A). You can get old exams from upper classmates, teaching assistants, or sometimes the professor, if you explain that most of the class has them. Hustling for old exams is a skill you should learn and constantly refine, since you'll need it later in medical school, where exams are even more repetitive and predictable.

Of course, this must all be done in the realm of honest, ethical behavior. Cheaters do not get into med school.

**2. Take a reasonable course load.** Another golden rule to success in college: don't overload your class schedule. Most students realize that if they had more time, they could do better in their courses. In other words, the problem is not that certain courses are intrinsically difficult; it's that they are time-consuming, and they take time away from all your other courses.

Don't get the wrong idea—we are not suggesting that you attend school part-time. Rather, we suggest you eliminate super-macho schedules. For example, some students think they can take four laboratory courses in one semester and still get a 3.7 GPA. If you can, more power to you, and we'll congratulate you when you get the Nobel Prize. However, most students get only poor grades and lots of stress.

A reasonable schedule means more time. More time means less stress. Less stress means you will enjoy the courses you're taking and think more deeply about them. It's ironic that, although a university exists to foster creative thinking, most students feel such time pressure that creative thought becomes nearly impossible.

**3. Study alone.** For most circumstances, we advise you to study alone.

Many people insist that group study is best because you're forced to think hard about the topic when you must explain it to someone else. As a result, they say, group study will expose weaknesses in your comprehension.

It sounds good, but most group study doesn't work out that way. Instead of quizzing each other and discussing topics relevant to the course, you spend a lot of your time gossiping about the party last weekend. If your study partner is attractive, you won't be concentrating on the material. Plus, there's usually somebody in the group who only wants to be tutored, and he's so far behind that he can't contribute anything. (He's usually the same person who asks you for lecture notes because he felt class wasn't as important as his sleep.)

Don't misunderstand—sometimes it is appropriate to form a group to tackle class material. If a professor is disorganized and confusing, a study session with good students can clear up tough concepts. And topics that require a lot of memorization are easier to learn if another person quizzes you (e.g., organic chemistry reactions).

But nine times out of ten, you're better off studying alone, without all the distractions of a group.

**4. Choose the proper study environment.** Study in a quiet place that's not too comfortable. Some people claim they can study on a couch while they watch MTV. For most students, however, this is the first step to disaster.

Courses like physics and chemistry require deep, sustained concentration, and distractions like TV and radio only hinder good studying. College life comes with many freedoms that can make grades suffer if a student can't impose self-discipline. Part of being a physician (or an adult, for that matter) is knowing when to work and when to play. Developing such habits early will make life much easier in the future.

A library-like environment is where you will study most efficiently. If you study on your bed, odds are you'll fall asleep. Unfortunately, many libraries are uncomfortable. You should find a quiet, comfortable place where you can think intensely for long hours.

**5. Highlight your books.** Students from most public high schools, where it is a capital offense to put even a light pencil mark in a textbook, may have a tough time with this. However, universities require students to purchase their own books, and usually at high prices. Since you own these expensive texts, it's totally acceptable and certainly advisable to write in them.

Highlighting is a good way to filter out minor details, and it's an excellent way to review for exams. If you don't write in your texts because you want to keep them in pristine condition, you're making studying much more difficult than it need be. Besides, the resale value of marked-up books is exactly the same as clean books.

**6. Make flash cards.** Most people do not like to use flash cards because it reminds them of learning multiplication tables in third grade. But flash cards are the most useful—and least used—study technique.

Flash cards appear to be expensive and time-consuming to make. This is true only if you wait until the end of a course to make them. We have found that folding a regular sheet of paper into sixteen squares and then cutting them out makes the best size (and least expensive) flash cards. Use paper clips to keep them in convenient bundles, and make them as you go along with your studies.

For instance, when you highlight a concept in a book, write it on a flash card as a question, with the question on one side and the answer on the other. Once you've made the cards, even material that involves simple regurgitation will be easier to learn. Since you already wrote them, the cards make reviewing the material as fast and as good, if not better, as being quizzed by another student.

**7. Keep a social life.** Although many college students tend to socialize at the expense of good grades, some premeds go to the opposite extreme and withdraw entirely from the fun of college life. But that's a mistake, because social relaxation provides an excellent release for tension and prevents burnout. Moreover, a moderate social life will actually enhance your academics. You'll find that wasting an evening at the movies or at the local tavern will put you in a much better mood to study organic chemistry the next morning.

A social life will keep your eyes open to the rest of the world and will remind you that there's more to life than the basement of the library. Your undergraduate years should be some of the best years of your life, so it only makes sense to enjoy them as much as possible.

**8. Understand concepts that seem unlikely to appear on the exam.**

Professors realize there are certain topics with which most students have problems. Many times we would say to ourselves, "He'd never test us on this stuff. It's too hard, and he spent only five minutes discussing it." Guess what? The obscure stuff would always be on the exam, and they were always the questions that most of the class got wrong.

Most professors write exams with a bell curve in mind: there are questions everyone should be able to answer, questions some people should be able to answer, and a few questions that only the top students will get. Topics that seem trivial and ambiguous are, as one professor told us, "excellent material with which to separate the A students from the B students."

Look at it this way: it's just a game, so be a smart player and pay attention to even the most minor details.

**9. Don't memorize when you can understand.**

If you can learn something by either memorizing it or conceptually understanding it, always choose the latter. Generally, it's less efficient to memorize many details than to understand a general principle from which you can derive the specifics.

Learning things this way will help you excel in courses like physics and chemistry, where exam questions are not identical to, but similar to, the homework problems. If you understand the principle well, you'll be able to apply the concept to the problem on the exam.

## *Improving Grades by Being Assertive*

Although studying hard is probably the single most important factor in achieving high grades, there are times when being aggressive may be just what it takes to push you from a B+ to an A-.

Unfortunately, some students take this philosophy to the extreme, and it only works against them. They are perceived as obnoxious, and teaching assistants and students avoid helping them. Some of these "grade grubbers" will argue for every little point on every exam. When it comes time for recommendations, you can bet professors tell medical schools about a grade grubber's real personality.

On the other hand, letting professors or T.A.'s get away with grading errors or unfairness is no good either. So, you should try to walk that fine line between being an over-aggressive jerk and being a piece of driftwood. By doing this, you can sometimes push your grade a little higher.

For example, don't be afraid during a lecture to ask the professor to explain a concept again. Better yet, ask the professor about it after class. It may turn up on the exam, and professors instinctively try to help students with material related to exam questions. When the student gets the question right, the professor feels he has done an excellent job teaching the material!

Also, get to know your teaching assistant. You don't have to be a brown-noser, but you should ask for help whenever you need it. If the T.A. sees that you're making a sincere effort, he'll be more willing to help you and may even boost your grade if you're on a borderline.

Finally, stand up for your rights. Tell your professors and or T.A.'s if you think they are out of line (e.g. giving what you think is a bad test, not spending enough time on a difficult concept, etc.). Don't threaten and don't whine, but talk to them in a rational, mature manner. You'll be surprised how interested they are in your opinion. They'll usually make changes or suggest ways you can overcome your difficulty.

## *Pass/Fail Grades*

An easy and enjoyable way to take a course is on a pass/fail basis. Unfortunately, competition for medical school makes taking your required premedical courses pass/fail unadvisable, because med schools have no way to interpret what a "pass" means in relation to your peers. Taking a few courses like sailing or drama pass/fail isn't a problem, but never take Organic pass/fail!

If you attend a college that uses a pass/fail system in lieu of all grades, request that your work be graded. It is unfortunate that stimulating learning experiences must be perverted into a scramble for grades, but that's the premedical reality.

# Chapter 3

# The MCAT

We cannot over-emphasize the importance of good MCAT scores. Though standardized tests continue to be criticized as culturally biased and dehumanizing, the MCAT remains the standard by which medical schools level grades from many different schools.

Nearly all medical schools require the MCAT. It's crucial that your scores be as high as possible, because at many med schools, only the combination of your grades and your MCAT scores determines whether you get an interview letter or a rejection letter. It's a very cold, objective, impersonal process.

The moral of the story is simple: Don't treat lightly something that may mean as much as—if not more than—three years of grades combined.

## MCAT Sections

The current MCAT consists of four sections, including a writing sample. The test lasts five hours and 45 minutes, but when you add a lunch break and the usual standardized testing delays, you'll be there about eight hours.

Section One of the exam, called **Verbal Reasoning** (a.k.a. "reading comprehension"), involves multiple-choice questions based on reading passages about 500 words long. The topics are selected at random from the humanities, social sciences, and natural sciences, and you're not expected to have any knowledge of the subjects.

People who usually do well on reading comprehension tests should have no trouble on this section. English majors, for example, will have a real advantage, since they have typically done more critical reading than the average science major. If you're anxious about this section, there's really only one solution: read more! One recent test taker suggested reading newspaper editorials, since their length and style approximate the Verbal Reasoning passages fairly well. But in the long run, you'll probably help yourself just as much by getting a good night's sleep and eating a light breakfast before the exam.

Section Two, **Physical Sciences**, consists of physics and chemistry questions. You're expected to answer the questions based on your knowledge of basic science concepts, plus your comprehension of the information presented in passages, graphs, and tables that accompany the questions. Unlike Section One, you can greatly improve your score in Section Two through intensive review of course material.

After lunch, you get Section Three, the **Writing Sample**, which requires you to write two essays, each based on a quotation. You have 30 minutes for each essay, and in each you must first interpret the statement, then oppose the statement, and then resolve the conflict you've established. The key to this section is to remember that the graders are only expecting a "first-draft" effort. Don't get caught with an unfinished essay because you've been rewriting, revising, and polishing your interpretation. It's far more important to complete the three tasks in an organized, coherent fashion.

Section Three is made more challenging by the fact that it begins right after lunch. Often, people finish Section Two feeling very hungry, so they gorge themselves at lunch. Then they return to the testing room and start to feel drowsy, suffering from what we call *food coma*! By the time they've got to write the second essay, their minds have turned to mush.

The remedy for this is easy: don't eat large portions of red meat or greasy food at lunch. Instead, eat trail mix, salad, fish, chicken, or other light fare.

If you don't stuff yourself during lunch and remain calm

while writing, you shouldn't have overwhelming problems with Section Three.

Section Four, **Biological Sciences**, is identical in format to Section Two, except for two big differences. First, the questions address biology and organic chemistry. Second, it's the last section of the test, and you'll undoubtedly be sick and tired of filling in those little bubbles with your #2 pencil.

The solution to the first problem is simple: study. The solution to the fatigue is a little sneakier. Bring something sugary, like a Snickers bar, in your pocket. (Technically, food is not allowed in the testing room, but who ever bothers with petty rules like that?) During Section Three, eat the candy. If you time it right, you should have a big sugar high to get you through the last section. So after the test you lapse into a food coma. But who cares? It's over!

It's important to remember that the MCAT is designed to break you and everyone else. The propaganda written by the test-makers will tell you that the MCAT will measure the "problem-solving" and "communication" skills necessary for your career as a physician. Maybe, but what it really measures is your endurance, which is probably the most important quality you need to be a doctor anyway.

With the MCAT you have no choice: you must play their game, by their rules. But you can play it smart. Everyone knows it's just a weeder, so don't get hyper-anxious and let yourself become a weed that gets plucked.

## Scoring the MCAT

The MCAT gives four scores, which reflect your performance in each section. The scores for Verbal Reasoning, Physical Sciences, and Biological Sciences are reported on a scale of 1 to 15 (with 15 as the highest). Your raw score—the actual number of correctly answered problems—is converted to this 1 to 15 scale so people who take different MCATs can be compared to one another.

In the Writing Sample, two readers grade each essay "holistically," which can be best defined as "by gut feeling." You don't get one point for spelling, one point for sentence structure, one point for grammar, and so on. Instead, readers give a single score for their overall impression of the essay. However, your score will be reduced automatically if you don't address all three tasks required in each essay. The four essay scores (two per essay) are combined into one raw score, which gets converted to an alphabetical scale of J to T (with T as the highest).

Although your raw score may be lower than the raw score of someone who took the MCAT after you, your scaled score may be the same, because it reflects your performance among your peers who took the test at the same time—and that's the truly useful data. The test makers do their best to offer equivalent MCATs from year to year. They adjust for the slight variations in each test-taking population by shifting the bell curve that corresponds to the scaled scores.

Many med schools look for consistency in MCAT scores. If your three numerical scores are above 10, and your essay score is respectable, your chances of an interview are quite good. But two 14's on the science sections won't help if you got a 6 in Verbal Reasoning and your essay score is appropriate for someone who drew pretty pictures on the paper.

Interestingly, studies have found little correlation between high MCAT scores and good medical school performance. And high grades in med school don't guarantee you'll be a good physician, either. But medical schools will continue to use the MCAT to make decisions about applicants, so you're just going to have to deal with it.

## *Preparing for the MCAT*

When you receive your MCAT registration packet from the Association of American Medical Colleges, you'll read on the second page of the instruction booklet something like, "The AAMC has conducted analyses comparing the performances of examinees who enroll in commercial review courses with those who do not (*yak, yak, yak, blah, blah, blah*), and we have found that gains derived from taking commercial review courses are small—only one-half of one scaled score point."

Now, this may sound like doing well on the MCAT has something to do with genetics or your intrinsic intelligence or something crazy like that. Well, that's simply bunk! The MCAT is not the SAT, and it's not about seeing three dimensional relationships in space, à la IQ tests. It's about knowing old concepts so well that they're as fresh as when you first learned them two or three years ago.

The point is, there are no curve balls on the MCAT, and studying for it, as for any other test, will boost your scores.

But there are no short cuts, either. Preparing for the MCAT requires a lot of diligence—and diligence is what the MCAT measures! Getting high scores is really a function of how badly you want to get in, and, in our opinion, how badly you want to get in is the most important information an admissions committee can have about your potential success.

The earlier you start preparing, the better. Reviewing for the MCAT will involve effort as any other test—just much, much more. We recommend you start the review at least six (and probably nine) months before the exam. This doesn't mean reading an MCAT review book five minutes before you go to bed. You should start an intensive review of concepts and information that will be pertinent to the exam (see outline in *The MCAT Student Manual*).

We cannot stress enough the importance of focusing your study on relevant topics during this critical period. For example, don't start reviewing old notes from chemistry class, because you'll only get bogged down in an incredible amount of superfluous material. You'll end up studying information in a depth that you'll never see on the MCAT. (By the way, this skill of discriminating study will be essential in medical school, where you must decide what's important from a mind-boggling amount of information.)

Remember, the MCAT tests very basic concepts. Occasionally they are disguised in a somewhat complicated question, but usually they are given in a straightforward manner.

The problem is, there are many questions on a wide range of topics, so you may be asking, "Well, how do I know what basic concepts to study and what to ignore?" Fortunately, someone has answered that question for you. Perhaps the most important investment you can make to get into medical school (besides this book, of course) is *A Complete Preparation for the MCAT: The Betz Guide* (formerly known by the name of one of its authors, Dr. James Flowers). The authors offer succinct review notes that parallel the outline of science topics in *The MCAT Student Manual*, which is written by the same people who devise the MCAT.

Get the idea? The authors imply that if you know the *Betz Guide* thoroughly, you should average a minimum of 11 on the science portions of the MCAT. From our personal experience, this is quite accurate.

Unfortunately, it's more difficult to increase your scores in the reading and writing sections, because they involve skills that you either have or have not developed in the course of your entire education. So don't sweat it! You can't worry about things you can't improve. Concentrate on what you most certainly can improve: your science scores.

## Professional MCAT Prep Courses

What about professional preparatory courses like Stanley Kaplan, Bar/Bri, The Princeton Review, etc.? We recommend them, but you should realize that you'll get out of them only what you put into them.

Stanley Kaplan Testing Centers offer the most popular courses. Now, we all know Stan makes big bucks every year off a lot a premedical students, but for about $800 he can do a lot more for your MCAT scores than $80,000 worth of private college will. Plus, his fee doesn't seem so large when you consider that you could spend up to $5,000 just applying to med school.

For most students, the in-class part of the Kaplan course is not worthwhile—they don't tell you anything you can't get on your own. What you're really buying are hundreds of simulated MCAT exams. Stan can go a little overboard with the depth of his exam questions, so if you're getting about 75% or 80% on his exams, you'll probably get 11's or 12's on the real MCAT.

We suggest you take all the Kaplan tests. Then, listen only

to the recorded answers of the questions you got wrong. Finally, review the subject areas that gave you difficulty in the practice tests. This process alone will take three months to do thoroughly. We can't guarantee you'll see identical questions on the real MCAT you take, but you'll have solved so many similar problems that it'll be a real challenge for the test-maker to write a question that doesn't resemble a problem you've already seen on a Kaplan test.

In any event, Kaplan's tests show you where you are weak, and they decrease your anxiety about the MCAT—probably their most valuable function.

Again, to get your money's worth from any prep course, take all the sample tests and review your preparatory booklets on a regular basis. Set aside a regular time each week for intensive preparation. If you do these things consistently about 20 hours a week and begin six to nine months before the exam, almost nothing can stop you from getting good MCAT scores.

As for the author's personal experiences: John studied Kaplan, became a believer and then an instructor. Dan also took the Kaplan course and did OK on the MCAT. Stephanie, on the other hand, regularly worked through the *Betz Guide*, aced the MCAT, and saved some money. Decide on the approach you think will work for you.

## Examination Tips

Though some of the following suggestions may seem obvious, students often forget them under the pressures of an exam. Therefore, read through them before you take the MCAT to remind yourself of test-taking strategies, and remember to adhere to them even when the test is not going smoothly:

1. **Read all directions with great care.** It's ridiculous how many errors occur due to carelessness in reading directions and headings.

2. **Time is a limiting factor.** Remember this when you're tempted to leave a question unanswered, with the expecta-

tion of returning to it later. The best thing to do is mark your best guess for the moment and star the question so you can go back to it later if you have time.

**3. Be conscious of your allotted time.** You must budget your time for each of the sections on the exam, so take a watch to the test. According to the *The MCAT Student Manual*, your total score is a reflection of your right answers only. This means you aren't penalized for guessing, so always guess! Never leave any bubbles blank. If you have 30 seconds left and 10 unanswered questions, just fill in the same letter (e.g., "b") for all of them.

**4. In the Verbal Reasoning section, quickly read the *questions* before you read the passage.** This way, you'll recognize the sections in the passage that deal with the questions. Also, the questions are usually in the same order as the information in the passage, except sometimes one question comes right away that you can't answer until you finish the passage. Knowing this, you can usually keep the next question in mind, read the passage until you come to the answer, and then move on. By doing this, you read the passage only once and save a lot of time.

**5. All questions in the Verbal Reasoning section are based only on information in the passage.** Do not use your own knowledge to answer any questions. Base your answers solely on the information in the passage.

**6. Before starting each essay, write a very brief outline in the margin of the booklet.** If you start to get bogged down in the essay, refer to the outline and recall the key points you want to express. If you try to organize it all in your head, you probably won't write a clear essay.

**7. While working the science sections, rely on your fundamental understanding of chemistry, biology, and physics.** Most questions in the science sections deal exclusively with basic principles.

# Suggested Reading

**Medical School Admission Requirements.** *Association of American Medical Colleges, Membership & Publication Orders, 2450 N Street NW, Washington, DC 20037-1129. Phone 202-828-0416.* **$10.** The Bible! New edition available each April.

**The MCAT Student Manual** (includes MCAT Practice Test I). *Same address as above.* **$15.** Do not take the MCAT without this one! It contains an authentic sample MCAT, which will give you an excellent idea of what the test is like and the kind of scores you'll receive. Also available: a second set of publications, including *MCAT Practice Items—Verbal Reasoning & Writing Sample, MCAT Practice Items—Physical Science & Biological Science*, and *MCAT Practice Test II* (an actual MCAT, administered April, 1991).

**Minority Student Opportunities in United States Medical Schools.** *Also at AAMC address above.* **$7.50.** Many special programs are available to minority students, and this is the official directory.

**A Complete Preparation for the MCAT: The Betz Guide.** *Betz Publishing Company, P.O. Box 1745, Rockville, MD 20849. Phone toll-free 800-634-4365.* **$49.50** plus $6.00 shipping. This is absolutely the best preparation for the science sections of the MCAT—and we don't even get a royalty for saying so.

# Chapter 4

# The Application Process

In the preceding chapters, we described ways you can achieve your highest potential grade point average and MCAT score. After you've followed these recommendations, the time will finally come for you to apply to medical schools, to show the various admissions committees why you should be allowed to enter their school. It is the most critical and, in some ways, the most difficult step.

You'll probably feel frustrated when you realize that you're expected to transfer years of preparation and effort onto four pieces of paper. While we agree this may not be the best way to evaluate an applicant, we are not writing a critique of the admissions process here. We just want to tell you how to work best within the system and how to make the system work for you. As far as admissions committees are concerned, you are *only* what your application says you are (until the interview), and you should use this fact to your advantage.

**The closest to perfection a person ever comes is when he fills out a job application form.**

**—Stanley J. Randall**

If admissions committees were able to live with applicants and see them as they really are, they'd probably reject most of them. So here's a flaw in the process that works *for* you: those four sheets of paper are not very good at revealing what a person is really like. With a little effort, anyone can shine on an application.

Often, applicants are unsuccessful simply because they haven't mastered the ability to manipulate the process to their advantage as well as others. Our goal is to refine your skills of manipulation.

The two components of your application that are already set in stone are your grade point average and MCAT scores. You can't change them, so don't worry about them. Your "personal statement" (usually a biographical essay) and recommendations are items that you'll complete shortly before you send your application. (The end of this chapter has a concise timetable of events in the application process. Use it to mark your progress and keep track of important events.)

If you already have good grades, don't write anything in your essay that could give a bad impression (e.g., extremist political opinions, embarrassing personal details, etc.). If your grades aren't so great, the essay is your chance to show what you're really made of. An excellent essay and glowing recommendations are the only items in the application over which you have control. Their careful execution is critical, and we will discuss them in greater detail shortly.

Remember, your application is the only "you" that medical schools will know. If they are impressed with the "you" on the application, they will want to see the real you for an interview.

## AMCAS and the Application

Years ago, applying to medical school was an even more laborious task. Students had to fill out a separate application for every school—a time-consuming process, as you can imagine.

Fortunately, the American Medical College Application Service (AMCAS) has simplified the process. You can now send one application to AMCAS, which will forward copies to the schools you specify. Unfortunately, a few medical colleges are still not part of AMCAS, and you must request separate applications from each of these schools. As of this writing, the non-AMCAS schools are

| Baylor | Texas Tech |
| Brown | U. Missouri, Kansas City |
| Columbia | U. North Dakota |
| Harvard | U. Rochester |
| Johns Hopkins | U. Texas (Dallas, Galveston, |
| New York University | Houston, San Antonio) |
| Texas A & M | Yale |

You'll find these schools' addresses in *Medical School Admission Requirements* (see page 35), which should be your Bible. It includes every essential piece of information on admission statistics and requirements you could possibly imagine. Get it. You will refer to it often.

AMCAS is just the first level of the application process. When you make it through AMCAS, you'll get a secondary application unique for each school. They range from a more detailed version of the AMCAS application to a simple request for more money "so we may further evaluate your application."

After the secondary application, you'll be asked for an interview. Rejection can come at any stage, but making it through AMCAS is the most important hurdle, because after AMCAS the process becomes a little more personal and subjective. It's easier to be "creative" post-AMCAS than in the pre-AMCAS, GPA-and-MCATs-only stage.

You can get an AMCAS application from your premedical advisor, from AMCAS medical schools, or from AMCAS directly at

> AMCAS
> Association of American Medical Colleges
> Section for Student Services
> 2450 N St. NW
> Washington, DC 20037-1129
> (Phone 202-828-0600)

Your application must include a check, which is AMCAS's fee for its distribution service. The amount depends on the number of schools to which you want your application sent. (For the 1995 entering class, the fee was $200 for six schools, and $10 for each school over six.) Then, the med schools will request about $50 extra when you receive their secondary application. You can get some of these fees waived if you can demonstrate financial hardship.

You must also send an official transcript to AMCAS of all college work completed. You should request this from your school early, since many large schools are slow, and the delay will hold up the rest of your AMCAS application. Most medical schools ask you to put your last semester's grades on the back of their secondary application, saying they "won't get the latest transcripts in time." Actually, it's a sly way to test your integrity. Any discrepancy between the grades you report and official records will prompt the admissions committee to reject your application immediately.

You will not need to send your MCAT scores, since AMCAS is the same swell bunch that gave you the MCAT. How nice . . .

Both the AMCAS application and the secondary applications have deadlines. A golden rule in this game is to submit every application at the *earliest* allowed date. Many people think medical schools wait for all applications, make their selections, and reject the rest. Nothing could be further from the truth. Students are accepted on a **rolling basis**. In other words, every day after the earliest possible date you wait to send your application, you have less and less chance of being admitted. Many qualified applicants have been shocked into reality when they waited until the last minute to apply and found that no spaces remained.

## *Your Extracurricular Activities*

Extracurricular activities are very important to your application—never believe otherwise—because they tell medical schools things about you that your GPA and MCATs never will. Of course, med schools first want to know that you're intellectually competent, but they also want to see more than just scores and a high I.Q. Extracurricular activities demon-

**A man may be so much of everything that he is nothing of anything.**

*—Samuel Johnson*

strate your personality, your motivation level, and even your basis for choosing medicine.

Before you say, "I want to be a doctor," it's crucial to know why you really mean it. Spending all your time making an A in Organic Chemistry will never tell you if medicine is your calling. Therefore, it's **imperative** that you go to a hospital and do some sort of medical work. If they won't employ you, then volunteer. You'll gain experience and knowledge, and you'll show medical schools that you're genuinely motivated and interested. When they ask, "So, Mr. Smith, why do you want to become a doctor?" you can say, "Well, for the past three years I've worked in an emergency room near campus, and I've found it rewarding and fascinating."

Similarly, if medical research is your thing, you can apply for summer work in a genetic engineering company or any firm engaged in biomedical research.

This way, you'll show that you've based your decision to enter medicine on practical, personal experience—experience that will impress admissions committees of the validity and conviction of your statement. (*Note:* Most committees actually assign points to applicants' files based on the breadth and depth of their medical-related work.)

The key concept is simple: get medical experience as an undergraduate, and make it your principal extracurricular activity. If you have an interest in a particular field of medicine, try to get work in that field. You might be surprised to learn that pediatrics, for example, isn't right for you after all. It's much better to find out early than ten years down the road, when it will be much harder to change professions.

If you don't have an interest in any specialty, don't be afraid to try anything in a hospital that will give you good experience. It may work out great, or it may bore you to tears. What's important is that it's a learning experience and a chance for you to check out the business, so to speak. Don't fool yourself by thinking that after you get accepted to medical school you'll have lots of time to decide what kind of doctor you want to be. You don't. So it's a good idea to start looking around in your college years, when making an incorrect choice won't hurt much.

If you can't find a position in a medical field that interests you, check a service-related field. For example, drug counselor, resident advisor, suicide prevention hotline volunteer, etc. are good options. Such activities indicate your desire to help people—a very important trait. Many applicants will talk about how much they want to "help humanity," yet their only extracurriculars are "fraternity social chairman" and "captain of co-ed water polo team." No wonder admissions committees treat them with skepticism.

Finally, extracurricular work totally unrelated to medicine may be fine also. If you do something that interests and intrigues your interviewers, you will stick out in their minds. After seeing 300 applicants, interviewers tend to view everyone as pretty similar.

For instance, if an applicant had average grades and MCAT scores and no relevant medical work—but she had won an Olympic medal—she'd probably land in medical school easily. Similarly, a college student who started his own pizza parlor or had a book published would also stand out from the pack. This doesn't mean you have to become an Olympic athlete or an entrepreneur. But if you want to do some kind of unique work, by all means do it. The main point: be interesting.

However, extracurricular activities should never come at the expense of your GPA. No amount of extracurriculars will be an excuse for poor grades. Also, it's not necessary for you to list thousands of extracurriculars on your application. A few impressive activities in which you are genuinely involved count more than a deluge of "So what?" activities.

By now, most of you probably are wondering what you can do *this year* to put on your application. Well, you literally can do hundreds of things. All schools have clubs. (But don't think that just because there's a premedical club you should join it. Medical schools are rarely impressed with them.) Join a club that applies to your major. Becoming a club officer always looks impressive because it shows leadership potential—an important quality for many physicians. Being an athlete is also great. Anyone who can maintain a schedule of rigorous practice and studying and still keep good grades deserves to be commended. A student government office is good for similar reasons. Community volunteer work always looks good. Help out at a soup kitchen or with a literacy program, or join Big Brothers/Big Sisters.

If your school does any research at all, you should be able, with a little effort, to start working with a professor in his lab. If you are really lucky and dedicated, you may even get your name on a publication. This is extremely impressive! You might even consider being a teaching assistant in a course.

As for summer work, many universities and their medical schools sponsor programs designed especially for the undergraduate who wants hands-on experience. It's no secret that many people are admitted to medical schools through "back doors" like these. The programs offer a great opportunity for you to work for, and get to know, someone on the med school's admissions committee. It doesn't guarantee you'll get in, of course, but a personal contact can't hurt. Medical schools will send you the relevant information on these programs, which often provide a stipend for living expenses.

Finally, if all you can do in the summer is work in a regular job (waitress, delivery man, working for your dad, etc.) because you need the money, then that's what you must do. Just be sure to make your reasons clear in your application.

## *Recommendations*

Letters of evaluation are one of the most important factors in the selection of medical students. Therefore, like the MCAT, you must not take them lightly.

Many applicants don't start thinking about recommendations until junior year, when they're due. Ideally, though, you should start to think about them from Day One of *freshman* year! Students also mistakenly assume that the person who writes your recommendation is going to write a good one. Instead, you must constantly think, "Do my professors really know me, or am I just another body in the classroom?" When the time comes to ask your professors for recommendations and they don't even know your name, you'll be in deep trouble.

> I don't care what is written about me, so long as it isn't true.
>
> —*Katharine Hepburn*

We all know the students constantly blathering in class—and everyone wishes they would just shut up. Well, those are people the professor remembers, too, so try to be like them—but don't be pushy and obnoxious to the point that you're remembered in a negative way. Simply be inquisitive and sound interested. Try to see your professors in their office hours and ask only a few questions to clarify major points in class. You may be surprised to find that the subject matter becomes more interesting when you force yourself to look at the material hard enough to ask intelligent questions. If your questions are intricate, save them until after the lecture. Your professor will be impressed by the depth of your understanding and appreciate your not interrupting the flow of the lecture.

Ask only "clarification" questions in class. Don't publicly correct the professor when he is wrong, but don't hesitate to do so later in the form of a question. He'll announce the correction in the next class and remember your brilliance in his recommendation letter.

A good recommendation should reflect more than just a casual acquaintance. It should also carry some weight—the more the better. You don't need to solicit Nobel laureates, but a little strategic thinking about whom you will ask can do wonders to enhance your appeal to medical schools.

A professor should be able to say more about you than, "She received a grade of A in my class." Therefore, when you ask a professor for a recommendation, ask first if he thinks he can write you a good one. Tell him to be totally honest. It's the only way to get an idea of what he'll write, since you should always request to have a closed file. (A "closed file" means you are not allowed to look at what was written about you. It's the only way to get honest, credible letters, since a professor is likely to be less candid if he knows you can read what he wrote later. This goes for both praise and criticism.)

Further, to give the admissions committee a more balanced profile, choose professors from different fields (i.e., don't get recommendations from only your chemistry professor buddies).

A recommendation from the professor with whom you do research is great because it might tell an admissions committee about your lab expertise *and* how well you work with others. A letter from the physician who oversees your volunteer work is also valuable, because it might describe how you deal with sick people. Sometimes, it's even a good idea to have a teaching assistant who knows you well write the recommendation, and then have the professor co-sign it (only the prof's signature gives the letter any weight).

Letters of recommendation from family, friends, medical students, and high school teachers are not acceptable. They only indicate poor judgment by the applicant.

In the past, it was common to ask a professor directly for a recommendation to send to medical schools. Today, that practice has been supplanted by a **composite recommendation**, where a premedical committee at your college drafts a letter of recommendation from letters written by people of your choice. This means that getting to know your premedical advisor is a very good idea. This also means that if the premedical committee can't write a good letter, it doesn't matter how good the rest of your letters were.

You can't do much about the composite letter, so don't worry about it. If the committee can't write well, your only consolation is that everybody else in your school is in the same boat. However, most composite letters include direct quotes from the professors' letters. The composite letter also ranks you in comparison to your peers in motivation, integrity, sincerity, and leadership. In addition, the letter usually begins by saying how "competitive this undergraduate institution is, and how hard it is to get good grades at this great school, etc . . ."

Because it's all so subjective, most admissions committees ignore the bull and go straight to the quotes. Therefore, you should strongly suggest that your premedical committee include such quotes—and even the actual letters from your recommenders.

In short, the composite method has pitfalls, but try to use it to your advantage, and never make an enemy. You never know who will serve on the premedical committee.

## Filling Out the Application

Since the application is your chance to tell medical schools why you are so special, give it a lot of extra care.

The first rule: type it neatly. Never use a dot matrix printer. In fact, many students actually pay to have their essay professionally typeset, but that's probably going overboard. A good laser printer will suffice. Dr. W. Edwin Dodson, Dean of Admissions at Washington Univ., advises that, since members of admissions committee "tend to be old and have presbyopia, a font size less than 12 points irritates the reader"—something you definitely don't want to do.

> **An autobiography usually reveals nothing bad about the writer except his memory.**
> —*Franklin P. Jones*

Rule #2: the application should be totally perfect. A simple typographical error may be reason enough to reject someone when there are thousands of applicants to weed out.

Finally, don't even *consider* having someone else write your essay, let alone paying for such a service. Such "professional" essays are always too good to be true and will certainly raise some eyebrows. They may get you some interviews, but if your verbal skills resemble a punch-drunk boxer rather than William F. Buckley, you'll be out! Anyway, after four years of sweat, is that *really* the way you want to get into medical school?

Don't forget all the jobs you've held in the past few years. Many applicants never include some jobs because they think only work related to health care is significant. But any job shows a willingness to work—a trait you'll need in abundance in medical school. Besides, leaving out miscellaneous work experiences may result in that section of the application looking very empty.

Further, you never know what the person who reads your application is looking for, so include all your jobs. A member of an admissions committee told us a story that illustrates this point: An applicant's essay made the student sound so arrogant that the admissions officer was just about to toss the whole thing. Then, he noticed that the student had worked a summer in construction. He wondered how someone so pretentious could do that kind of job. Intrigued, he decided to interview him. It turned out the student wasn't at all the way he sounded in his essay, and he was admitted.

You should also include all the honors you've received. Many people initially think they have no honors, but when they think harder they realize they have a few awards to write in. Remember, never leave a section blank.

The key thing is, you're supposed to tell your life story on the application. In other words, you're describing how you spend your time. If you spend time climbing mountains, playing the flute, ballooning, singing opera, skydiving, surfing, or anything that's just plain out of the ordinary, let them know. Medical schools always like to say how interesting and diverse their students are. They just love it if you do something eccentric or unique—and you probably do if you think about it for a while.

## How Many Schools Should You Apply To?

Applying to medical school can be very expensive. You must pay for the AMCAS application, the secondary applications, and then transportation and accommodations when you interview. But compared to the cost of a medical education, the application expense is trivial, and you should never let money limit the number of schools to which you apply.

**There are three kinds of lies: lies, damned lies, and statistics.**

**—Benjamin Disraeli**

If you can demonstrate financial hardship, you can get the AMCAS (and sometimes the secondary application) fees waived. However, most students do not fall in the extremely low family income level that's required for a waiver, even though you may be receiving financial aid at college. Often, medical schools will help reduce your expenses by letting you stay with a student when you interview.

But even after cutting lots of corners, you're still looking at a cost somewhere between $1,000-$5,000, depending on how many schools you apply to. That may sound outrageous, but consider what your undergraduate education will cost— probably $30,000-$100,000—then add the potential cost of med school—another $60,000-$100,000. Compared to this, even a large application budget is fairly insignificant.

Therefore, it doesn't matter whether you must beg or borrow—you should *never* let financial matters become a limiting factor in your application to medical school. Years of expensive work and planning should not go down the drain for such a minor reason.

So the question becomes, "How many schools should I apply to?" There's no easy answer, but consider the following: The average medical school receives about 5,000 applications for 100 positions. If the selection process were entirely random, your chance of acceptance would be one-in-50 (2%). To put it in a more depressing way, your chance of rejection would be 98%. Sounds pretty dismal, doesn't it?

But wait. If you apply to a number of schools, your chance of being accepted by at least one school is one minus your chance of being rejected by all of the schools. That is,

$$\% \text{ ACCEPTANCE} = 1-(.98)N \times 100$$

where N is the number of schools to which you apply. Let's plug in some sample numbers:

| N= | % ACCEPTANCE |
|----|----|
| 1 | 2 |
| 5 | 10 |
| 10 | 18 |
| 20 | 33 |
| 30 | 45 |

In reality, of course, the process is not totally random, though there are random elements in it. The point is, even if you're a straight-A student, it would be unwise to apply to fewer than five schools. Basically, the more the better. If you are a really strong student, you should apply to no fewer than ten. If you're like most people, 20 and even 30 schools would be a good idea.

Many applicants don't realize that applying to as many schools as possible is as important as doing well in school or on the MCAT. Of course, you must never compromise quality for quantity of applications.

The 2% probability of acceptance at a particular medical school is not really as bad as it sounds. In the 1993 entering class, 42,808 applicants applied for 16,307 places. So, your actual overall probability of being accepted to at least one medical school (if you apply across the board) is about 40%. Not bad. The figure of 2% comes from the fact that every applicant applies to more than one school, giving the illusion that there are more applicants than available positions. Therefore, your chance of being accepted to at least one medical school after applying to 20 is actually higher than 33%, because the number of applicants is much less than the number of applications received by medical schools.

Our goal here is not to turn you into a statistician or a gambler, but to stress the point that all the hard work in the world won't get you in if you don't apply intelligently. You must be fully aware of how to increase your odds—which usually means submitting as many applications as possible. As Dean Dodson advises, "Apply early; apply often—like voting in Chicago."

## Deciding Where to Apply

Students with high grades and MCAT scores will likely have a wide choice of medical schools to attend. However, they are a minority, because most students usually get accepted to only one or two schools. Therefore, it's critical that you choose the correct schools to which to apply.

We recommend that you divide the number of schools

you plan to apply to into quarters and rank them on their relative appeal. (The end of the chapter has a ranking of schools.) The first quarter should include schools where you never expect to get accepted but would attend instantly if you did (e.g., Harvard). The second quarter should include the very competitive schools, then the strong schools, and the final fourth should be all the rest.

For example, if you apply to 20 schools, you would choose five schools from each of the four groups at the end of the chapter. By spreading yourself out like this, you'll increase your odds of acceptance and maybe get some nice surprises.

You should consider whether the school is public or private. Of the medical students starting in 1992, 68% attended schools in their home state. In general, public schools accept mostly state residents, so applying to the Univ. of Tennessee when you live in Connecticut could be a total waste of time.

On the other hand, such a rule can work to your advantage. In some states, especially in the Midwest, the number of in-state applicants is so small that the public medical schools have trouble filling their classes. Therefore, nearly every state resident who applies gets in, so the admission requirements are much lower than at private schools. If you move to one of these states and establish residency, you have an almost sure acceptance to the state medical school. Of course, this ploy is drastic and should be a last resort.

Another thing to determine is the school's acceptance ratio (how many students it accepts versus how many apply). Of course, you'll want to look for the largest ratio. *Medical School Admission Requirements* will have all this data.

Other important questions to consider:

1. **Do you like the location?** Although you'll probably attend whatever school you get in—and you should never eliminate schools in your home state—it doesn't hurt to at least consider location before applying. There are many medical schools in many different locales, so you shouldn't have to settle for a place where you'll be miserable.

2. **What are the clinical and research facilities like?** This is very important, because it will give you an indication of

what types of patients you'll see and how many you'll see. In general, county and city hospitals see much more action, courtesy of the local "knife and gun clubs," than private hospitals. The number of patients the hospital treats annually will also indicate how much clinical experience you'll get. If you want to become involved in research, find out the amount and type of research conducted at that school.

3. **How is the education delivered?** Find out how many days per week—and how many hours per day—you're in school. Most medical schools go five days a week; some go four or six. Some have nine hours of class per day; others average only four. Some schools provide note-taking services; others make you struggle on your own. Some ease the tension by having a pass/fail grading system; others can be cutthroat and neurotic with letter grades. Interactive software, hypertext, and virtual reality are making education more fun at some schools, including Loma Linda, U.C. San Diego, N.Y.U., and Cornell. The curriculum may not seem important to you now, when all you're thinking about is "Will I get in?" but these points are critical, because they can make the difference between an exciting learning experience and an awful one.

4. **What about housing and health benefits?** High-quality, low-cost dormitories or subsidized housing can greatly affect your overall expenses, especially at urban schools. Living in a cockroach-infested apartment won't help your study habits much, either. Make sure to see the "typical" student housing and determine if housing is guaranteed for all four years. Health benefits are an important but often overlooked issue. Students are not employees and are not covered by employee health and disability programs. For instance, will prophylactic AZT be available in the event of an HIV-infected needle stick? Does the school provide the hepatitis B vaccine free? On a more mundane level, will you have to spend your hard-earned student loan money on dental work or contact lenses?

# Financial Aid for Medical School

It sounds implausible, but it's true: your finances should not restrict your choice of medical school. Once you are accepted, the school will work with you to ensure that you and your family will be able to pay tuition and still live well.

All medical schools inform students about the Stafford Loan program (formerly the Guaranteed Student Loan), Health Education Assistance Loan (HEAL), Supplemental Loan for Students (SLS), Perkins Loan, Homan Loan, University Loans, and other state programs. Note also the federally-funded Armed Forces Scholarship and the Medical Scientist Training Program (MSTP)—it's open to all and pays tuition plus stipend (see below for details). First- and second-year minority students should get information about the National Medical Fellowships.

There are many more scholarship and loan programs—too many to list here. The bottom line is, your medical school's financial aid office will help you meet the high cost of your education.

Don't worry too much about signing for loans, either. Despite the fact that the average total debt for 1992 med school graduates was over $55,000, you'll eventually be able to repay the loans for your tuition pretty easily. Skeptical? To convince you, we've listed below the 1991 nonacademic median salaries of the various specialties, as reported in the *Physician Compensation Survey Report* by the Center for Research in Ambulatory Health Care Administration and the Medical Group Practice Association:

| Specialty | Median Compensation |
| --- | --- |
| Anesthesiologist | $220,800 |
| Cardiologist (invasive) | $258,875 |
| Cardiovascular surgeon | $420,090 |
| Dermatologist | $145,092 |
| Emergency medicine | $123,942 |
| Family practicioner | $101,876 |
| Gastroenterologist | $188,133 |
| General surgeon | $172,952 |

| | |
|---|---|
| Internist | $110,606 |
| Neurologist | $132,000 |
| Neurosurgeon | $338,692 |
| Ob/Gyn | $197,745 |
| Orthopedic surgeon | $274,255 |
| Pediatrician | $104,937 |
| Psychiatrist | $110,143 |
| Pulmonologist | $154,795 |
| Radiologist | $246,462 |
| Urologist | $195,715 |

Since we have raised the issue of earning potential, we feel we should remind you that good medicine always requires the doctor to place the patients' needs first. If your goal is to make a ton of money in as little time as possible, go into investment banking. You'll be happier and society will benefit more. If your concern is how you're ever going to repay medical school loans, relax. There's no denying that you may face a short-term financial struggle, and you may have to wait a little longer than your business school friends to buy a house or vacation in Hawaii. But if you're enjoying your profession, it's well worth it.

## Final Review of Your Application

A few more points to consider before you mail that AMCAS application:

1. **Make a final check for absolute, 100% neatness.**

2. **Have other people read what you've written.** Your premedical advisor, a premedical friend, or the family physician are good choices, since they are familiar with the process. An English teacher can help with style or grammar problems.

3. **Make sure you use the entire space** (with reasonably sized print and margins, of course) for personal comments, and try to be original. For example, don't write about how

you've wanted to be a doctor since you were a kid. This was everyone's ambition at age four. Most applicants will spend months working on their essay before they write the final version, so get started way in advance. We'll discuss the essay in greater depth in Chapter 6.

4. **Photocopy the application** and keep it in a safe place in case AMCAS loses it, and also for interview preparation.

5. **Always send the application via certified mail** if you are approaching a deadline. This will put the burden of explanation on AMCAS should the application be lost.

## After You've Applied

Once you file your application, it will be just a matter of time before you receive requests for interviews. In the meantime, it's important that you follow up on your application.

For starters, keep a meticulous record of your status at each school. We recommend making a chart with your schools in one column and receipt of application, secondary application, interview, etc. in other columns. Write in the date when each category is filled. This way, you'll know if a school seems overdue for a note or phone call from you.

It's perfectly acceptable to phone schools. Of course, you don't what to harass them, but calling occasionally to determine the status of your application is a good idea, since applications do get lost and letters of recommendation misplaced. If you try to be extremely cordial on the phone, you may find yourself on a first-name basis with the secretaries. This may sound unimportant, but one applicant got to know the secretary well enough that she hand-carried his application to the Dean of Admissions at U.C. Davis. The fax machine can be another very useful tool.

If you're not accepted right away, don't panic and ruin your senior year of college. Some applicants will receive acceptance letters in the fall, but don't expect to be accepted until the spring.

Often, half of an entering medical class comes from the

waiting list, so don't get discouraged if you are wait-listed. If several schools do put you on a waiting list, the odds are good you'll get into at least one, since these lists are usually about twice as large as the actual entering class.

As you wait to hear from schools, have an answering machine or someone always available to receive messages, especially as you approach the end of summer and the beginning of medical school registration. Be sure to notify the schools if your address or phone number changes.

Also, keep the admissions department abreast of any new awards, publications, etc. that may strengthen your application. (However, sending new transcripts, unless they are dramatically improved, is usually not helpful.) Here's a good example: A student had planned to matriculate at his second-choice school. The week before classes began, he was in the newspaper for placing third in a balloon race in Allentown, PA. He mailed the article to his first-choice school and drew an arrow to himself in the newspaper photograph saying, "Please, pick me up!" The school called him the day before classes began and offered him admission. After partying on Bourbon Street in New Orleans, he sped north to New York City—another happy ending . . .

## *Handling Acceptances*

Students usually begin collecting letters of acceptance at their safety schools first. According to the rules of the game, applicants may not hold more than one acceptance offer after May 15. If you're waiting to compare financial aid packages, make sure to contact the schools involved and apprise them of this before the deadline.

This rule can make things tricky. For example, one applicant was holding acceptances to four schools when a Director of Admissions threatened to retract his acceptance if the applicant didn't decide soon. (All AMCAS-participating schools know your status at the other schools to which you applied.) After being confronted, the student rushed to the post office and declined admission at three of the four schools. For the fourth school, he quickly filled out and mailed the registration form weeks early—thereby committing himself to that school.

A few days later, Johns Hopkins (a better school than any of the original four that had accepted him) learned that the applicant was now holding only one spot, and they offered him a place. Unfortunately, Johns Hopkins had to retract the offer when they discovered that the student had officially registered at another school.

The lesson: don't hold multiple acceptances, but don't rush to register at any school early.

## *Special Programs\**

**Medical Scientist Training Program (MSTP):** The National Institutes of Health (NIH) provides funding to students who wish to pursue scientific and medical training (M.D.-Ph.D.) at the 31 schools listed below. Each year, approximately 140 new students receive scholarships that pay a stipend of $8,800, plus full tuition. In 1992, 806 MSTP students were supported by the federal government. After training, the student is obligated to conduct research or teach, usually for five years.

Another 112 schools provide the option of obtaining a combined M.D.-Ph.D. degree, but these are not funded by the NIH. Some of these programs are funded privately; others are not funded at all. Information on these programs usually comes with the school's application.

The NIH-supported programs are at these schools:

| | |
|---|---|
| Albert Einstein | UCLA |
| Baylor | U.C. San Diego |
| Case Western Reserve | U.C. San Francisco |
| Chicago-Pritzker | U. Iowa |
| Columbia | U. Michigan |
| Cornell | U. Minnesota |
| Duke | U. Pennsylvania |

---

*Data from *Medical School Admissions Requirements, 1993-94*, published by the Association of American Medical Colleges.

Emory
Harvard
Johns Hopkins
Mount Sinai
New York U.
Northwestern
Stanford
SUNY Stonybrook
U. Alabama

U. Pittsburgh
U. Rochester
U. Texas, Dallas
U. Virginia
U. Washington
Vanderbilt
Washington U. (St. Louis)
Yale

**B.A./B.S.-M.D. Programs:** A few medical schools offer select high school students the opportunity to combine their undergraduate and medical training. The program, usually six years, lets students avoid much of the anxiety of the medical school application process. Two of the programs—SUNY-Stonybrook and UMDNJ-Robert Wood Johnson—select students at the end of their sophomore year in college. Some programs operate in combination with several undergraduate colleges.

Albany Medical College
Boston U.
Brown
Case Western Reserve
Chicago Medical School
East Tennessee State
Hahnemann (Philadelphia)
Howard (Washington, DC)
Louisiana State-Shreveport*
Medical College of Pennsylvania
New York U.
Northeastern Ohio
Northwestern
Penn State

UMDNJ—Robert Wood
  Johnson
SUNY Brooklyn
SUNY Stonybrook
Thomas Jefferson
  (Philadelphia)
UCLA
U. Miami
U. Michigan
U. Missouri, Kansas City
U. Rochester
U. South Alabama
U. Wisconsin, Madison

*Program limited to state residents.

**M.D.-J.D. Programs:** This combined program allows medical students to pursue a law degree as well as an M.D. The following schools offer this program:

| | |
|---|---|
| Chicago-Pritzker | U. Illinois at Urbana-Champaign |
| Duke | U. Pennsylvania |
| Southern Illinois U. | Yale |

## *Timetable of Important Dates*

### JUNIOR YEAR

#### NOVEMBER THROUGH APRIL:

❑ Begin review for MCATs.

#### FEBRUARY OR MARCH:

❑ Apply for spring MCAT.

#### APRIL:

❑ Think about which medical schools to apply to.
❑ Collect letters of recommendation.
❑ Suggested time to take MCAT.
❑ Get the AMCAS application packet from your premedical advisor or request it from

*American Medical College Application Service*
*Association of American Medical Colleges*
*Section for Student Services*
*2450 N Street NW*
*Washington, DC 20037-1129*
*Phone: 202-828-0600*

#### MAY:

❑ Interpret MCAT scores and GPA with premedical advisor (see note below).
❑ Make first draft of AMCAS essay.

❏ Send for medical school catalogs.
❏ Send transcripts to AMCAS and non-AMCAS schools.

### JUNE:

❏ Revise and polish AMCAS essay.
❏ Submit AMCAS application at earliest allowed date.
❏ Begin completing non-AMCAS applications as soon as possible.

### AUGUST:

❏ Inform premedical committee where to send your composite recommendation letter (if your school has such a committee)
❏ Register for fall MCAT if scores were low and you feel you are now better prepared.

## *SENIOR YEAR*

### SEPTEMBER:

❏ Make sure that your applications are complete and that letters of recommendation have been received. Call to confirm if necessary.
❏ Fall MCAT offered.

### NOVEMBER:

❏ Be patient. Interviews will come!

### DECEMBER:

❏ Try to schedule interviews during Winter Break for convenience.

### JANUARY:

❏ Fill out GAPSFAS form for financial aid.
❏ Send updated transcripts if requested by schools.

### FEBRUARY:

❏ If no one loves you by Valentine's Day, speak imme-

diately with your premedical advisor. He or she may
be able to call on your behalf.

❏ If you are wait-listed, send a letter expressing continued interest.

❏ Acceptance letters are still sent out, so stay calm.
Make sure medical schools can reach you or a family
member by telephone at all times.

Note: Keep in mind that a few undergraduate programs
like to boast "our acceptance rate to medical school is 80%"
because it sounds impressive to high school students. (That
is, students are more willing to pay the high tuition the
school demands because they think they'll definitely get into
medical school from that college.)

In reality, the acceptance rate is so high because the school
does a student weed-out. They tell mediocre students that
their chances of getting into medical school are horrible, so
they shouldn't even apply (when in fact they may have a reasonable chance of acceptance). So the only students who
apply are stars who will get in easily—thus giving the high
acceptance rate.

The lesson here is simple: take your premedical advisor's
counseling with a grain of salt. The ultimate decisions
should be yours alone.

## Breakdown of U.S. Medical Schools

The medical schools below are divided into four categories
to help you make a rational decision about which schools to
apply to. (Schools in Groups II and III are alphabetized within the group, not ranked.) The groups are based on ratings
from *The Gourman Report* by Dr. Jack Gourman (National
Education Standards, 1993). For further reference, consult
the March 21, 1994 issue of *U.S. News & World Report*.

## Group I: Most Competitive

1. Harvard Medical School
2. Johns Hopkins University
3. University of Pennsylvania
4. University of California—San Francisco
5. Yale University
6. University of Chicago
7. Columbia University
8. Stanford University
9. Cornell University
10. University of Michigan
11. University of California, Los Angeles
12. Duke University
13. New York University
14. Northwestern University
15. University of Minnesota
16. Tulane University
17. University of Rochester
18. Washington University, St. Louis
19. Vanderbilt University
20. University of California, San Diego

## Group II: Very Competitive

Baylor College of Medicine
Boston University
Bowman Gray School of Medicine
Emory University
Georgetown University
George Washington University
Indiana University
Loma Linda University
Ohio State University
State University of New York at Buffalo
Tufts University
University of California, Davis
University of California, Irvine
University of Illinois
University of Iowa

University of North Carolina
University of Pittsburgh
University of Virginia
University of Washington
University of Wisconsin

**Group III: Competitive**

Albany Medical College
Albert Einstein
Brown University Program in Medicine
Case Western Reserve University
Creighton University
Dartmouth Medical School
Health Sciences University, Portland
Loyola University of Chicago
Mount Sinai
Saint Louis University
State University of New York at Stony Brook
Temple University
University of Colorado
University of Connecticut
University of Kansas
University of Louisville
University of Maryland
University of Missouri, Columbia
University of Southern California
Wayne State University

**Group IV: Good**
Most everything else.

## The Nation's Best Hospitals*

| | |
|---|---|
| Johns Hopkins Hospital | Baltimore, MD |
| Mayo Clinic | Rochester, MN |
| UCLA Medical Center | Los Angeles, CA |
| Massachusetts General | Boston, MA |
| Cleveland Clinic | Cleveland, OH |
| Duke University Medical Center | Durham, NC |
| UCSF Medical Center | San Francisco, CA |
| Brigham & Women's Hospital | Boston, MA |
| Barnes Hospital | St. Louis, MO |
| Columbia-Presbyterian Medical Center | New York, NY |
| Memorial Sloan-Kettering Cancer Center | New York, NY |
| Stanford University Hospital | Stanford, CA |
| University of Michigan Medical Center | Ann Arbor, MI |
| University of Texas (M.D. Anderson Cancer Center) | Houston, TX |
| University of Washington Medical Center | Seattle, WA |

*According to U.S. News & World Report, July 12, 1993.

# Chapter 5

# The Interview

For applicants with good grades and MCAT scores, the interview is often just a formality. But for most students, it is a critical part of the admissions process.

The purpose of the interview is to obtain information independent of and supplementary to the data you supplied on the application. An interviewer may assess a candidate's academic potential, maturity, motivation, leadership, interests, knowledge of medicine, attitude, ability to relate to others, and other subjective criteria. A strong interview can increase your chance of admission tremendously, and a bad one can destroy even the class valedictorian. Therefore, it's essential that you understand the ingredients of a good interview.

**The real art of conversation is not only to say the right thing in the right place, but to leave unsaid the wrong thing at the tempting moment.**

**—Dorothy Nevill**

We believe interviewing is a skill you can learn. But, of course, it's impossible for us to teach you through a book. Improvement requires personal interaction. For example, if you think you may come across as shy, arrogant, or whatever, ask a friend or your premedical advisor to conduct mock interviews with you. It's an excellent way to improve your interviewing skills.

Better yet, use a video camera and VCR to study yourself as you answer questions. The tape will give you a realistic picture of how others perceive you. There are even courses designed to teach interviewing skills, but don't bother taking them unless you have a major problem (e.g., extreme shyness) to overcome.

## The Interview Process

In general, the interview process is divided into three parts: the orientation, the tour, and the actual interview.

Not every school offers an orientation, but most do. Its purpose is not to evaluate applicants, but to inform them about what the day will entail.

All the other applicants to be interviewed will be with you at the orientation. Some may try to give you the impression that they are totally superior or that they were Albert Einstein in a past life or something. Don't pay any attention to them. They're just playing mind games with you and trying to mess with their competition. Just remain pleasant and smile a lot. Your display of maturity will probably bug them more than anything else you could do.

Use the orientation as a time to relax and gather your thoughts. Remember, if you are asked for an interview, it means they want you as much as you want them. Their goal for that day will be to sell you on their school and convince you to attend it over other schools that might accept you.

## The Tour

After the orientation, you'll tour the medical school. The tour, which will cover the clinical and instructional facilities, is when you'll get the big sales pitch. Many applicants get so anxious about their interview that they forget that the *school* is really the one under scrutiny. Contrary to popular opinion, one medical school is not like the next. Each has a unique personality, which you may or may not like.

A medical student who has no bearing whatsoever on admissions decisions usually gives the tour, so feel free to ask any questions. It's essential that you take time in the tour to get a feel for the school, in case you must decide between two or more schools.

For this reason, unless lack of funds totally prohibits travel, never accept the option to be interviewed in your area rather than at the school. Many schools send a representative to, say, California to interview applicants who can't afford (or just don't want) to fly east.

If you can, spend the night before the interview with a medical student. He/she will usually offer good insight about what things are really like at the school.

## *The Interview*

Your interviewers will usually be two faculty members or one faculty member and one medical student. In the latter case, the faculty member will carry more weight, but don't underestimate the input from the student. Acting like he/she is a peon in the admissions process will guarantee your rejection. The faculty interview may help you get in, while the medical student interview can weed you out.

Again, either or both may be on the admissions committee, so it's not a good idea to say anything too bizarre. Instead, the interview is your chance to expand on information that may not be clear to the committee. Applications do not have enough room for detail, and they force the applicant to abbreviate and oversimplify. Just remember to be yourself, since it's usually easy for an experienced interviewer to tell if someone is lying or exaggerating.

Some schools turn the interview into a contest. At Northwestern and Emory (or so the rumor mills report), a few students are lined up and interrogated as a group by a panel of admissions officers. Although this can be an intimidating and somewhat impersonal situation, you can benefit by using the time when other applicants are talking to formulate a better response of your own.

Many people tell horror stories of how a "friend of a friend" had some doctor give a him a really hard time in an interview. Of course, it's possible you'll encounter a jerk, but most interviewers want to make the experience as stress-free as possible. Don't forget—the interviewer has been through the same thing and will be aware of (and usually sympathetic to) your nervousness.

One of our classmates did have a real hard time in one interview. At the end, the doctor said, "Sorry I was so hard on you, but it's only because I really want to recommend you. I wanted to be sure you had the right stuff. If I don't want somebody, I usually just give him a real easy interview."

So don't try to judge what somebody thinks of you by the way they treat you in the interview. Sometimes, they just want to see how you react to a stressful situation.

For example, there's an interviewer at a Texas school who shakes your hand, smiles, and asks, "So, how many times a week do you masturbate?" A friend of ours answered, without missing a beat, "Not as much as I deserve." Another friend was asked, "So, when are you going to get married?" To which she replied, "Is this a proposal?" Yet another female friend was asked, "Once you get married, how will your husband feel about your palpating another man's scrotum?" Her reply was calm and professional.

Interviewers ask such questions only to see how you react to very personal or taboo subjects. Reacting with humor or maturity is far wiser than getting angry or upset. Remember, a physician must handle complex moral and ethical issues—and all types of patients—in a dignified, tactful manner.

Then there are interviewers who just like to hear themselves talk. They want to impress you with how much they think they know. All you have to do is be a good listener, seem interested, and be patient. It'll be over soon.

Finally, if you don't know an answer to a question, just say, "I don't know." Nothing sounds worse than someone fumbling to make up an answer.

## Final Preparation before the Interview

You probably know the cliché, "You only get one chance to make a first impression." And given the volume of applicants that interviewers must see, the first impression is often the *only* impression. This means that for men, a suit, and for women, a conservative dress or suit, are mandatory. And don't neglect grooming. Get a haircut, trim your beard, clean your fingernails, etc. We don't mean to sound like your mom, but the informality of dorm life at college can make you forget how people dress and behave in the real world.

Before the interview, review your photocopy of the application you sent to the school. Often, interviewers will ask you to clarify or elaborate on something in your application. Chances are, you filled it out two months ago, and if you don't review it beforehand, you probably won't remember what the point was. This looks bad.

Also, read the catalog the school sent you. Having a little substantive knowledge about the school looks impressive.

Above all, remember to pronounce the interviewer's name correctly, since you'll want to say, "Thank you, Dr. Radiziewski. It's been a pleasure speaking with you," or whatever. No sound is more important to people than the sound of their own names. In medical school interviews and in life in general, always refer to people by their names. It makes them feel, consciously or subconsciously, important—and they'll remember your kindness.

Being polite and personal also helps with the secretaries in the admissions office. More than one applicant has been derailed by being rude to the secretary. The secretary often attends the final admissions committee meeting, and since she has met all the applicants, she may occasionally make a negative statement—guaranteed to sink that student. No medical college wants someone who brown-noses professors and physicians while treating nurses, secretaries, and administrators with contempt. Besides, being on a first-name basis with the secretaries can help tremendously when you are curious about the status of your application.

## Sample Interview Questions

Your interviewers will ask a variety of questions, and your answers should demonstrate your maturity, character, knowledge, and ability to communicate. There's really no way to "study" for an interview, but for curiosity's sake, we've compiled a list of questions asked in actual interviews. You may not get similar questions, but it might be useful just for practice to think about how you would answer them.

How do you know that medicine is for you?

What has been your most important accomplishment?

Do you think doctors are viewed with as much respect today as in the past?

Is medicine becoming more technical, and is this beneficial?

What do you think of euthanasia? Abortion?

What can be done about rising health-care costs?

If a 15-year-old girl comes to you and wants birth control pills, what would you tell her?

How do you feel about animal research?

What do you think about the current push to limit the number of specialty residency positions?

Tell me about your research work. *(Be sure you understand thoroughly any lab work you've participated in, no matter how small your role.)*

What are your strong points? What are your weaknesses?

Do you have any hobbies?

Are you interested in any specialties?

What will you do if you don't get accepted to medical school?

Why do you want to work with sick people?

Do you think doctors are overpaid?

Do you feel you are prepared to enter medical school?

Why did you apply to this school?

What other schools did you apply to? Why?

How will you finance your education?

Tell us about your undergraduate institution.

When did you decide to become a doctor?

Would you consider applying to a foreign medical school if you were rejected by all the U.S. schools?

Are quotas fair?

Are you concerned about the surplus of doctors that's supposed to occur when you begin practicing?

What makes you different from everyone else?

What do you know about AIDS? How do you feel about treating HIV-positive patients?

What three adjectives best describe you?

What do you see yourself doing 10 years from now? *(A very popular question. Unfortunately, one student answered, "Uh, this is Wednesday, about two o'clock, right?" The interviewer said, "Yes, it is." The student swung his arm up as if he were holding a golf club and said, "I should be on the eighth hole." Apparently, his humor wasn't appreciated—he was rejected by that school.)*

Where would you go to medical school, given the choice?

How do you intend to integrate medical school (or your medical practice) and your family/social life?

What do you do for fun?

Describe your relationship with your family.

What do you know about hospices, HMOs, or PPOs?

How do you think malpractice will affect you?

What do you expect to get from medicine?

Do you have any children, or plan to? *(This is actually an illegal question, because female applicants are asked it far more often than males. But this is not the time to start quoting the law. Just give a straightforward answer, and try not to act offended.)*

What questions do you have? *(You could ask: What do you think are this school's weaknesses and how are they being improved? What research opportunities would I have? How is your school unique? How would you describe the typical class personality here? and so on.)*

# Chapter 6

# The Essay

So, your transcript is complete, the MCAT is over, and you are now completing the AMCAS application. At this point, your immediate goal is to get an interview.

As we have already noted, some applicants will be rejected immediately because their scores and grades are too low, while others are almost guaranteed interviews because of their amazing numbers. For students between these two extremes (probably most of you), nothing is stamped in concrete, and a good essay can earn an interview. On the other hand, an excellent applicant who writes a sloppy essay or a weird piece about how his parents are pressuring him into medicine may in fact be writing his own rejection letter.

Everyone has an image of "the good physician," and, fair or not, you will be measured against this image. While ambition and intellect are important, the committee is also seeking students who are compassionate, sensitive, and committed to medicine. Your essay should help the interviewers develop this image of you, and you can expect them to read your essay before the interview or immediately afterwards.

Following this chapter are actual AMCAS essays by medical students accepted at Cornell, Johns Hopkins, Yale, Harvard, Columbia, Univ. of Pennsylvania, N.Y.U., Washington University, and other top schools. We believe these pieces will give you a feel for the creativity and self-description that infuses a successful essay, and we hope they will be a catalyst for your own creativity.

We have intentionally mixed exceptional essays with more ordinary pieces to illustrate a simple point: even applicants with mediocre essays get into top medical schools. Of course, you should try to model your essay after the best presented here. To help you, we will comment briefly on the strengths and weaknesses of representative essays.

## *Authorship, Proofreading, and Style*

This section addresses two important points. First, the ideas and writing style should be all your own! If you have not internalized a philosophy of medicine—and developed a coherent way of expressing it—it will show in the interview.

Second, your message is more important than your writing style, but don't make a bad impression with convoluted prose and sloppiness. Deans of Admission assume your essay was proofread by Mom, Dad, a professor, a premedical advisor, and six or seven roommates, so don't hesitate to ask someone to check at least your spelling and grammar.

Essay #1 is extremely well written. The applicant clearly communicates her ideas and convinces the reader she has thought maturely about her goals. You can bet the interviewer asked her more about her view of life and her experiences with hematology/oncology and counseling.

The writing style in Essay #19 is unique. It shouts the applicant's enthusiasm and excitement about entering medicine and enjoying life. He takes the reader on a trip to the ocean, classroom, kitchen, subway, frat house, forest, and physician's office. He does not follow another's path or force himself into the premedical mold. Rather, he presents himself as a naturalist, idealist, and romantic.

If the writer of Essay #2 had not been accepted to medical school, she could have made a living as a book or movie critic. The beginning of the essay conjures vivid images of the doctor and disease, and we are left feeling that the applicant is the humanitarian. In fact, we feel she is talking about herself when she writes, "through close reading, the author's philosophy of life can be discovered." Not only does she recognize the value of a liberal arts education, she personalizes her view of medicine.

The best essays attract attention with an opening sentence that grabs the reader, draws him into the piece, and ties together the rest of the work. In journalism, it's called a "good lead." Examples include

Essay #45—"If you don't get paid, why the Hell do you work here?"

Essay #27—"A successful and effective physician must possess two essential qualities—a thirst for knowledge, and a deep motivation to aid his fellow man."

Essay #33—"What kind of person would be insane enough to spend half of his life studying for a job which requires twelve hour work days, no vacations, and interminable patience—in other words total dedication?"

Essay #41—"**Praeludium**. In the beginning there was dissonance."

A good lead puts readers on your side and makes them want to read more. It also makes your essay memorable.

Rather than being a hodgepodge of thoughts and achievements, your essay should also have a central theme or motif to bridge experiences, concepts, and extracurricular activities. The author of Essay #8 uses "communication" to discuss nature, philosophy of medicine, and life experiences. With society criticizing medical schools for producing impersonal robots, a poet who communicates well will stand out from the crowd.

In contrast, Essay #20 exemplifies a subtle mistake in many essays: Applicants begin their essays with an interesting concept, question, or idea, only to stray from the central theme when listing personal achievements. As a result, the body of this essay does not clearly support the lead or the conclusions. If at all possible, list your accomplishments elsewhere in the application, or have them described in your letters of recommendation. Use the essay for more personal communication.

Once you've written your final draft, there are only a few conventional standards to follow when typing your essay. Most important, be neat! Check that there are no visible corrections or spelling mistakes. This may seem obvious, but we were shocked at the number of typographical errors. Normally, applicants use a word processor or pay to have the essay professionally typed.

The length of the essay is variable. Of the essays we reviewed, some were short, such as Essay #11 with fewer than 200 words and #45 with fewer than 400 words. At the other extreme, #41 exceeded 1,500 words on one page. A successful essay does not have to fill the entire page with print. It's better to express your feelings and drives succinctly. (*Brevity is the soul of wit.*—Thoreau)

There is also no consistency among essays as regards margins, spacing, paragraphing, or print type. At the bottom of Essays #39 and #46, the applicants typed and signed their names. This adds a personal touch and authenticity, and may be appropriate for some.

In sum, the successful essay comes in all shapes and sizes, but its appearance and style is not nearly as important as its message.

## *Conservative and Safe*

A conservative and safe essay can still succeed. The author of Essay #21 recognizes that many of the people who will be reading his essay are academic physicians. Saying that he eventually wants "to work in a university affiliated hospital, and to be involved in clinically related research, while maintaining patient contact" is exactly what they want to hear. He stresses he is excited about the field of medicine and believes he will enjoy caring for the sick. He mirrors his reader.

Having stressed the "correct" reasons for entering medicine, he then fills the essay with information and details that are probably interesting to the researcher and impressive to the layman—but they add little (good or bad) to the picture of the applicant as a person. Early in his career, this student apparently decided to follow the Hippocratic Oath: *Primum non nocere* ("Above all, do no harm").

Often, the committee member is looking for students with a sense of balance between humanities and sciences, course work and athletics, work and fun. As an undergraduate, the applicant in Essay #26 balanced "a full dose of the humanities *and* a strong foundation in the physical sciences"—he majored in both physics and English. The woman in Essay #42 shares, "I also enjoy both listening to and performing music and hope to strike a rewarding balance between personal and professional creativity." In Essay #17, no one could question the applicant's research background. He has published two papers and four abstracts—well above the norm. Further, his proficiency in science is balanced by his artistic talent, national tours, and Broadway performances.

Again, we stress that medical schools are not seeking obsessive/compulsive students willing to lock themselves up in a lab for days. Rather, the admissions committee looks for the well-rounded applicant.

The student in Essay #5 conservatively plays the premedical game well: she worked with disadvantaged children, balanced science studies with humanities courses, conducted research at prestigious places, and gained clinical experience. She does not directly say she is a "nice" person with "nice" qualities. Instead, she compliments physicians as caring, dedicated, and intelligent. Her essay boosts the ego of the reader—and subtly implies that she shares these attributes. This indirect method is successful.

## Creative Vs. Weird

A creative essay captures the reader's attention with humor or a startling oddness. Since an interviewer reads dozens of essays in one sitting, you want your essay to be remembered—but it must be remembered in a positive way.

Effectively using dialogue, the author of Essay #9 shows he has thought about his goals in clinical medicine and at the laboratory bench. He is inquisitive and motivated, and he realizes there's more to life than straight A's.

Essay #41 won't be forgotten. Written as a piece of music,

the paragraphs are divided into "Praeludium," "Allegro ma non troppo," "Andante," "Adagio," and "Allegro con spirito." Our only comment on this essay echoes what the King of Austria told Mozart after a performance: "This opera has too many notes."

In your effort to be original, do not come across as being weird or eccentric. Skirting the bizarre, Essay #36 states: "The stories that most appeal to me are of individuals alienated from, or cast into, an alien society, struggling to assert their independence and individuality. By suspending my disbelief, I can partake in the struggle of the fictional characters and feel their victories and defeats." The applicant recognizes that he is challenging psychological norms and continues, "I am careful, however, not to confuse my love of adventure and fantasy with my reasons for wanting to be a physician." However, we wonder whether he would have been so bold if he knew that admissions committees often ask psychiatrists to interview applicants who write anything unusual in their essays. Take heed.

## Apologetic, Egotistical, Doubtful, or Boring

As a rule, don't use the essay to apologize for a low grade or a less than perfect MCAT score, as in #11 or #39. Nobody is perfect, and admissions committees don't want a litany of excuses. They're looking for good reasons to accept you, not trivial reasons to weed you out. Instead, use the space to present positive information about yourself.

Essay #16 comes across as somewhat egotistical, and it exemplifies what *not* to write. There's no question the student has expertise in the lab, and his knowledge of AIDS makes him an attractive candidate. But a commitment to patients should be foremost—and in the first paragraph, not the last line. He should have emphasized his concern in a positive way, not the negative "I will not divorce myself from patient care." He constantly places himself first, and though that may be a characteristic of many ambitious people, it doesn't make for a sympathetic essay. He expresses "realistic concerns for the safety of myself" and anxiety about the

AIDS virus appearing in his own low-risk group. He says his greatest satisfaction is in the lab—before he mentions the plight of the AIDS patient. Twice he boasts about receiving strong recommendations and being the only student approved to enter his lab.

Obviously, this applicant has a lot going for him, but his essay is a real turn-off. With a little perspective—that is, put yourself in the *reader's* shoes—you can appear talented and positive without being arrogant. Allow your credentials to speak for themselves.

One essay we reviewed made a mistake by ending, "The school that accepts me will receive an excited student who will prove to the board of admissions that they did not make a mistake." Although the student wants to leave the committee with the message that he is "excited" about medicine, the reader instead is left wondering why it would be a "mistake" to admit him. What does the applicant feel he has to "prove to the board of admissions" after the fact? Maybe if your entire application is strong, the question is irrelevant, but if there's a weakness in your application, leave it alone.

A mature, appropriate sense of humor never hurts. In Essay #29, the author stresses how his knowledge of biological sciences will be useful when studying "*Neisseria gonnorhoae*." Whether intentional or not, it's a funny prediction. On the other hand, Essay #24 is amusing in the way the author sets the reader up by mentioning impressive accomplishments achieved in the past and possibly reached in the future. He then matter-of-factly presents unachievable personal goals. Amuse the reader and you will be remembered.

## Why a Physician?

Why you decided to become a doctor is a common essay theme. Some students always knew they wanted to be physicians, in the same way children decide they want to be a fireman, a teacher, or President of the United States. The applicant of Essay #39 states that she knew as a child she would be a physician when she grew up, and she discusses how her decision was logically reaffirmed over the years.

However, not every physician chose medicine as a kid playing with a toy stethoscope. Essay #34 typifies how most students shape their goals. This applicant mentions how his experiences as an E.M.T. on an ambulance crew and rescue squad were "invaluable training for a career in medicine." Some students, on the other hand, discuss the influence of literature on their decision to pursue medicine. In Essay #3, the student is inspired by Doctor Dolittle and Charles Darwin, while the author of Essay #2 is influenced by a character in *The Plague*.

Professional paths are best decided with maturity and insight. The applicant of Essay #22 began bird-watching in college, had a gut feeling he would enjoy medicine, and tested his interest with clinical, research, and volunteer experiences. He has a good feeling for what lies ahead: "The science may interest me, the diagnoses may challenge me, but it will be that personal involvement with the patient that will make the most difference to me and keep me going through the hardest parts."

## Translating Research into Clinical Practice

In general, the most prestigious medical schools emphasize basic research. While only a handful of students actually pursue academic medicine, almost all successful applicants have at least token laboratory experience.

In your essay, you may choose to mention what you did, where you worked, and with whom. In any case, you will want to stress how much you enjoy research (embellish if necessary).

For example, in Essay #33 the student recalls "an incredible high" when his first scientific paper was published. The student in Essay #40 states, "In the long run though, I would like to be a physician who researches medicine on a 'basic science' level and, at the same time, translates advances in scientific theory into clinical practice." Likewise, the applicant in Essay #42 concludes, "I would therefore gain satisfaction from involvement in both the research aspect of medicine and its practical applications in patient care."

Don't panic if you haven't done lab work. You can still mention your dream of pursuing (time permitting) the Nobel Prize in Medicine. And if you aren't convincing, remember that research experience is neither required nor expected at less competitive institutions. Some applicants can get accepted without ever spending a weekend with a pipette, flask, or bunsen burner.

If you really enjoy research, consider the M.D.-Ph.D. programs listed at the end of Chapter 5. If selected, you receive a nice stipend, and your education is completely paid for. (Mom and Dad will love that.) When applying to an intensive joint program like an M.D.-Ph.D., be sure your essay shows balance. Don't discuss research for 99% of the essay, and then give one line to medicine. Remember that biomedical research, treating patients, and teaching are three equally important aspects of academic medicine. Essays #10 and #17 make this point well. Nonetheless, the author of Essay #11 is an M.D.-Ph.D. applicant, and his essay addressed only academics (and briefly), but worked.

## Meeting the Physician Shortage

Most medical schools actively recruit qualified minority students who express an interest in serving segments of the population that don't have access to excellent medical care.

In Essay #6, the applicant, a Mexican-American, has considered practicing in a needy Latin American country. He expresses altruistic motives, and he shows scientific aptitude with his authorship on a published paper.

The student in Essay #38 had his interest in medicine sparked after participating in the American Foundation for Negro Affairs Program. Later, he worked in a hematology department testing for sickle cell anemia.

The applicant in Essay #29 states, "My ethnic background has been a contributing factor in my prospective plans after medical school. I would like to work in a physician shortage area where my Puerto Rican background will be helpful in dealing with other Hispanic minorities." She believes it is her "duty in life" to care for others. Essay #43 was also written by a Hispanic who has worked with the poor.

Women as a group have been underrepresented in medicine. Since medicine has been a male-dominated profession, the female doctor sometimes confronts sexist attitudes. The woman in Essay #32 states, "Medicine was a serious consideration but due to the conservative attitude of my parents and Switzerland, the idea of a woman in medicine was not well supported." More alarming than parental pressures are the many female applicants who tell the story of a male doctor who asked during the interview, "Won't your career be ruined when you have a family?" (But remember, he may only have been trying to rattle them.)

The applicant in Essay #10 has insight into the concerns of many admissions officers about the role of women in medicine. She has chosen to confront sexism by describing a successful woman/physician/scientist who also has a happy family life. The applicant feels she can balance her profession and personal life, and she addresses the issue up front.

Older students often have gained skills and knowledge in fields that might further medicine. One applicant we know attended Bible college and wants to become a missionary doctor. The applicant in Essay #46 pursued a Ph.D. in psychobiology. We also know students who worked as investment bankers, teachers, scientists, police officers, and even medical school professors before beginning med school.

Admissions committees do not expect applicants to know for certain the field of practice they will enter. However, if you think you want to work in an under-served region or less-popular specialty, say so. The minority student in Essay #7 wants to improve health care for the indigent and the elderly. His interests in academic medicine and public health are admirable, because they are areas of medicine criticized for lacking dedicated physicians. He acknowledges that he has benefited from special opportunities made available to him, and now he says he's eager to use his background to help society. This applicant also improved his chances for admission by participating in a summer program at his first-choice medical school while applying.

Good medical care is also lacking in many rural areas,

where the applicant in Essay #12 wants to practice. She describes how her goals developed and how her interests are consistent with her goals. With admissions committees knowledgeable about the problems facing rural areas, they would be hesitant to toss this application into a rejection pile.

Other areas of physician shortage include primary care, public policy, armed forces, pediatrics, oncology, and geriatrics. Essays #26, #27, #29, and #34 express interest in these fields of practice.

## *Stamina*

In the past, endurance was extremely important for medical school admission, and a physical handicap would completely eliminate a student's chance for admission. Today, although most of our classmates are in good physical shape, some have speech, vision, or other disabilities.

Athletic involvement is a measure of physical stamina — and, presumably, your ability to withstand long nights in the emergency room. Essays #24, #32, and #44 all describe athletic exploits that indicate physical strength and a well-rounded person.

Mental stamina is equally important, and the admissions committee often respects a tough academic major. This probably accounts for engineers having such good luck with admissions. Essays #31, #35, and #38 were written by engineers. The applicant of Essay #38 already applied his skills and developed various prosthetics. And don't forget other challenging undergraduate majors, as in Essay #40. Statistically, economics majors fare well, too.

In addition to physical stamina and academic rigors, mental outlook is an important indicator used by the admissions committee to assess an applicant's fitness for medicine. In Essay #33, the student shares how asthma has influenced his life and decision to become a physician. The applicant in Essay #30 mentions his father's battle with schizophrenia and how the son matured because of the tragedy. In Essay #42, because the applicant witnessed the death of family members, she felt compelled to do her part to integrate modern science with medicine. Similarly, the applicant in Essay #48 was motivated to pursue medicine after helplessly watching a person die.

Witnessing illnesses and deaths are powerful influences. How you cope with tragedy is very much a part of the everyday life of a doctor.

Admissions committees will gain a sense of how you deal with the stresses inherent in medicine by how you respond to other types of adversity or pressures (as in the interview). The applicant in Essay #13 does not falter after a negative college event, but turns it into a positive, motivating experience. (*Note:* Just because the AMCAS application states that the applicant needs to explain any disciplinary action during college, don't assume you should devote the whole page to details. It's better to mention what you learned or how the adversity has helped direct you.)

## The M.D. Family

Sons and daughters of physicians pervade the medical school class. Historically, this is consistent with the Hippocratic Oath, which instructs the doctor "to regard his offspring as equal . . . and to teach them this art—if they desire to learn it."

Moreover, doctors' kids know what they're getting into. They know about the stress and its toll on the family. Children of physicians have a more realistic view of medicine, its practice, its demands, and its rewards.

Essays #18, #25, #26, #37, #44 were written by children of physicians.

## Name-Dropping

If you work for someone you know and respect, chances are he or she has many other friends as well. Essays #10, #28, #33, #42 describe by name their role models.

The physician in the first essay, for example, was known and liked at many of the medical schools to which the student applied. The applicant told us that once she learned that the interviewer and she had a mutual friend, she relaxed and did much better in the interview. It's easier to impress someone who already has a good reason to like you.

Likewise, the applicant in Essay #32 says her husband is at Cornell. Having a spouse at a medical school may help gain the applicant an interview. Med students often write letters on behalf of their spouses, boyfriends, or girlfriends. With a strong applicant, a letter of support may convince an admissions committee that the student will matriculate if offered acceptance. The alternative is a student who might transfer to another school later to join his or her spouse. Admissions committees dislike losing students to other schools and feel guilty about breaking up a family or romance.

The point is, if you have an inside connection, make it known to the committee.

Besides using personal contacts, some applicants will name the school they want to attend in their essay. We think this is a very risky tactic, but the applicant in Essay #46 knows where she wants to go: "I have chosen the Cornell Program due to its newly established PET facility as well as its exceptional reputation in the neurosciences."

We caution that name-dropping may limit your options. Presumably, the candidate in Essay #15 planned to attend Buffalo, Baylor, or Cornell. Experience and the contacts she made working at these schools give her an edge, but unless you are determined to attend a particular school, don't name-drop. Medical schools won't want to send an acceptance letter to someone they'll probably lose to another school. Remember, you must convince each school that it is among your top choices.

*A personal story from Daniel:* Many interviewers will ask, "What schools have you interviewed with?" Well, one school that interviewed me was SUNY Buffalo, where the interviewer asked me point-blank which school was my first choice and why. I was tempted to lie and say Buffalo, but I straddled the fence. "I am very interested in Buffalo," I replied, "but I would consider Cornell if I had a choice." After a while, he let me change the subject.

At the end of the hour, he studied my application again

while he made me wait for what seemed like an eternity. He then closed my file, tossed my application onto his desk, and said, "Mr. Jones, I do not think you'll be coming here."

*I really blew it!* I thought. I felt I had nothing to lose, so I challenged him. "What do you mean?" He explained that he thought I'd get into Cornell with no problem. He seemed to overlook that I had not yet interviewed there—a fact foremost in *my* mind. I reminded him that I liked the people I had met at Buffalo, that I thought the tuition was reasonable, and that I didn't mind the weather. In the end, Buffalo did accept me, but the doctor was right. I got into Cornell.

The lesson: doctors aren't stupid, and the interviewer will know you're lying—or at least being insincere—if you say you're dying to go to Podunk Medical School instead of Yale. So don't lie!

## A Word of Warning

As you read the essays, you might be tempted to highlight good lines and incorporate them verbatim into your own essay. Some students, unfortunately, might even want to swipe the whole piece and just "change it around a little."

We hope you realize how incredibly dumb that would be. Most admissions officers have read this book and these essays, and they would never admit a plagiarist. Any doubts about your integrity will destroy your application and your reputation.

## About the Essays

When you sit down to write your personal statement, we hope you'll use the essays as a catalyst to your creativity. As you read them, we think you'll be relieved to learn how broad the stylistic range is and how diverse the "acceptable" topics are.

The essays should also assist you as you consider your motivations for entering medicine and try to explain them. We cannot stress enough how important it is to be able to articulate your goals during the interview.

Each essay is reprinted exactly as it was written on the application. We have not corrected grammar, punctuation, or spelling errors. But note that rarely would such corrections be necessary. Occasionally, we have changed proper names and locations to guarantee anonymity.

Finally, we would again like to express our gratitude to the generous young doctors who allowed us to reprint their essays.

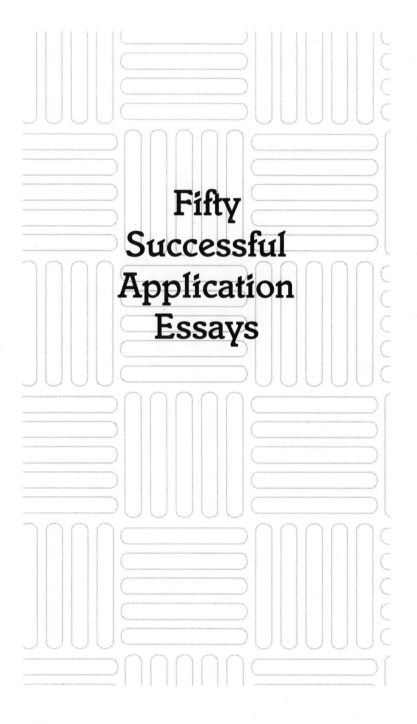

# Fifty
# Successful
# Application
# Essays

# Essay #1

My mother has told me that as a child my favorite question was "how come?" Rarely content with a simple explanation, I seemed constantly to have pushed my parents to give me more details about the way the world worked. This inquisitiveness, while sometimes the subject of affectionate joking, was always encouraged, even when answers were not available. I learned to value the explorative process as much as any "answer" found, and spent much of my free time discovering meadows and brooks, building imaginary civilizations, or immersing myself in a book. My parents are both English professors, and their love of the humanities has always been a vital part of my life. Although my exposure to the sciences at home was limited, I avidly pursued any outside opportunities to learn about the scientific world, and during my high school years the excitement of scientific discovery began to surpass any previous intellectual experiences I had had. Continuing with the humanities, I began to discover that for me novels and music were a luxury, offering pleasure and release. The happiness I derived from them did not have to be forsaken, but could be continued while I pursued a career in science.

Entering Wesleyan University, I thought I would major in Biology while simultaneously exploring as many other fields as possible, but my actual career goals were still hazy. I had previously acquired a taste for scholarship when I worked at Williams College as an archival assistant, but the somewhat solitary nature of the work had lead me to question my desire for a career devoted exclusively to research. During my first two years at Wesleyan, I took several laboratory corses, and found that although they were extremely time consuming, I was excited by the way classroom concepts came alive in the laboratory. Towards the end of my sophomore year a possible career in medicine first became a reality for me. Much that I valued seemed to be present within this field: the opportunity to acquire scientific knowledge, to do research, and to work with and help people. Seeking summer work that would give me the opportunity to explore medicine and medical research, I was fortunate enough to obtain a position in the Department of Hematology/Oncology at UCLA Hospital, with Dr. Martin Cline.

I am still awed by what occurred that summer. At nineteen, I walked into one of the most exciting and meaningful sectors of research in the country. The discoveries that were made while I worked in Dr. Cline's lab were extraordinary, and because I was an integral part of the functioning lab, I felt like an explorer myself. Since part of my responsibility involved getting cancer samples from the hospital every day, I also spent some time in the operating room and a lot of time in pathology. The exposure to clinical and surgical work was as valuable and stimulating as the research. The work was fascinating, the challenge a bit frightening, but I soon felt at ease in both lab and hospital. All that I had learned seemed to come miraculously together that summer.

The doctors I worked for became my mentors. I had not previously realized that one could be both a clinician and a research scientist, and while I sensed that research alone would not fulfill my needs, I still felt a desire to explore this option further. I looked forward to the research I had arranged to do at Wesleyan on my return. At the same time, however, I wanted more experience working directly with people, and when I went back to school in the fall, I trained to be a "listener" for 8 to 8, a student-run counseling service.

My junior year has been thoroughly enriched by my research and counseling experiences. The 8 to 8 training process was invaluable. Through it I learned a lot about myself—my attributes, faults, and values—and about human psychology. Working for the counseling service has strengthed considerably my conviction that medicine is, for me, an ideal vocation, one that would allow me to unite my scientific interests with the personal satisfaction I gain from helping and working with people. The research I am conducting at Wesleyan has been equally fulfilling. As my research experience has grown, my thought processes have slowly begun to change. Designing experiments, I have realized, requires foresight and a thorough integration of many concepts learned in the classroom, abilities I think are important for a doctor to possess, and that I hope I can continue to develop. This summer, at Brigham and Women's Hospital, I will again be doing research, and look forward to exploring still further the world of the laboratory.

My research experiences have been wonderfully rewarding, and I hope to continue laboratory work both through and after medical school. Clinical practice, however, is fundamentally more important to me, because it brings together my interest in people and my scientific and humanitarian ideals. I feel thoroughly committed to a career in medicine and only hope that I am able to give the profession as much as I think it can give to me.

# Essay #2

The narrator and hero of Albert Camus' novel, *The Plague*, is a doctor named Bernard Rieux. Amidst the horror of the plague which grips his city, the bureaucratic ineptitude, the religious fanaticism embraced by one character and the bleak existentialism presented by another, Dr. Rieux emerges as an advocate for the strength of human will and love. While the epidemic strikes people dead at random, rendering the efforts of medical science impotent, Rieux refuses to succumb to the belief that life is meaningless and tirelessly fights the plague with what little means he has. Romantic as this scenario sounds, Camus presents it objectively, and the novel's power lies in its almost journalistic reality.

When I read *The Plague* in high school, I was greatly drawn to the characteer of Rieux because of his humanism and because in the face of the epidemic he as a doctor was the only one who could actively do anything, though not much, to combat the disaster. The impotence which he felt against the plague is what all people must feel against any disease, although in many cases medicine can help a great deal. I had some contact with disease and injury while volunteering at a children's hospital in Cleveland. The patients ranged in age from two to twenty, and I visited them in their rooms, played games with or read to them, or just talked. I was glad to be able to give some emotional aid, but I felt powerless to change their condition. The dynamic power of medical science seemed very appealing to me during that experience.

However, as Camus illustrates through Dr. Rieux, being a physician involves more than scientific knowledge and its application. True sympathy—the ability to place oneself in the position of another—is what Rieux achieves and is what makes him a great doctor. I feel that studying literature is one of the best means of expanding one's sympathy. Not only does reading literature require an immersion in the emotional world of the characters, but through close reading, the author's philosophy of life can be discovered. This interpretation is what makes literature so challenging; the ideas are often not explicitly defined. I decided to major in English because I wanted an opportunity to study literature in depth and be able to discuss it with classmates and professors.

In addition to literature, I have taken many history courses, which I feel are equally as important to a liberal arts education. Knowing history helps one to place current social issues in perspective. Most of the history courses I have taken touched upon issues relevant to medicine and society. In an English history course, for example, I read about physicians in the eighteenth century who stole corpses from the gallows for anatomical dissection, because the supply of cadavers for research was strictly controlled by the government. The outrage of witnesses to this practice is paralleled by current public concern about the ethics of medical research, especially in the field of genetics. In my American history courses we covered topics ranging from the unrecognized outbreaks of malaria and typhus which killed many of the first settlers at Jamestown, to the establishment of Medicare under Lyndon Johnson. Studying history makes one aware of the tremendous advances in medical science, and also of the continuity of human attitudes towards medicine.

My own belief that humanism is vital to being a physician was reinforced during the summer I spent working in the Euclid Clinic. I helped patients settle their accounts and fill out insurance forms, so I had a great deal of patient contact. Most of the patients I saw had come directly from a doctor's office, and many of them wanted to talk about their visit. A frequent complaint which I heard was that their doctors rarely took time to listen to questions and worries, or give explanations and reassurance. The patients felt a need to tell someone about their illness or injury, and I spent a lot of time listening. My experience that summer left me with the feeling that although scientific skill may be the most important quality in a doctor, it is not the only necessary quality.

# Essay #3

I want to become a physician to heal people and to further my study of man as both creative thinker and purely biological animal. I think I've always been sensitive to the needs of others, and my experiences of the past few years have indicated to me that as a medical doctor I can make the progressive social contribution that is one of my life goals.

As a child I was preoccupied with things biological. I remember digging patiently among ants in their tunnels and trying to locate the eggs, capturing different bees from flowers, attempting to raise bird chicks fallen from their nests, and poring over slides of my blood and hair with a small microscope. Once I learned what the word meant I fancied myself a naturalist, and took great pleasure in the observations I made in the woods and marsh near our home. My favorite childhood books were Hugh Lofting's *Doctor Dolittle* series and Daniel Defoe's *Robinson Crusoe*. Later I read about Charles Darwin and John J. Audubon.

In high school I excelled in science subjects and was placed in advanced courses; I also concentrated on English and foreign languages. There was time for playing on the soccer team, practicing the cello, and writing for the school and community newspapers. I became more aware of chronic social problems, and passionately so. I took the AP courses in history and studied the evolution of man's endeavors to solve those problems. I discovered distinctions between various interpretations of objective history and visions of the future. I realized that while advances in technology were necessary for progress, their proper application was an equally important and complex issue. Technical advances in medicine, for example, are in themselves amazing but their utility is subject to ethical and economic considerations.

I viewed college as an opportunity for experimentation as well as for the pursuit of my established interests. I became interested in health care specifically while volunteering in the local Cerebral Palsy clinic. Our group worked primarily with young people in a weekly swim/gym program. I met on a regular basis with two boys who shared an uneasy friendship and were eager for attention from an adult. Once established, our relationship was a source of pleasure for me as well as for them. Hospital work in later years confirmed my positive attitude towards dealing with sick and handicapped people. Though I took premedical courses at Williams College, I was not intensely career-oriented. I wanted a broad education and chose history as its foundation. For my junior year I sought an experience outside the "ivory tower" of Williams. I attended the London School of Economics & Political Science, whose highly specialized curriculum complemented my more diverse program at home. Stimulated by the emphasis on independent work, I immersed myself in the study of modern history.

Following graduation from Williams I received a grant to serve as field assistant with a research team studying the physiology of the Black Rhinoceros in Kenya under the auspices of Harvard and Nairobi Universities. We worked with the Kenyan Game Dept. in moving the rare animals from highly poached areas to safer ones. Our group had access to the temporarily captive rhinos in order to record physiological data relevant to thermoregulation studies.

The rhino project ended in Sept. '80 but I stayed in Kenya to work with an ecologist doing a study of the carrying capacity for elephants in Meru National Park. When herds are confined to limited areas, their feeding destroys the vegetation quickly, and an aspect of large game management is determining the population a park can support. For a rapidly growing nation like Kenya, the problem is real; people are hungry and have little sympathy for animals that leave the parks to eat their crops. Actually I found the human side of the issue to be crucial; as both our needs and technology grow, so does our potential environmental impact. Development programs including a rational allocation of resources have become necessary to provide for both the "manmade" and "natural" worlds.

Medical care is one especially important part of the development strategy I'm referring to and is the focus of my interest. All through Kenya, Sudan, and Egypt I was amazed at the success of medical clinics that have, in fighting infectious disease, helped to raise birth and survival rates and life expectancies—but not necessarily the quality of life! More children survive into adulthood only to suffer from chronic malnutrition. Yet impoverished parents often rely on their children for security and disregard government urgings to limit family size. I feel that lay health education is an important adjunct to medical care programs.

The two years I spent in Africa and the Middle East experiencing vastly different cultures and living conditions have given me a new perspective here at home. I also gained confidence from dealing with accidents and other difficult situations that I hadn't encountered in school. I feel strongly that I have the potential for personal as well as professional growth in the study and practice of medicine.

# Essay #4

At the age of six I started studying insects under my magnifying glass and by the time I was ten, I had already detonated my first explosive with the help of a Mr. Wizard chemistry kit. These are just the first entries in my scientific resume. In high school I became more serious, studying the areas of electronics and meteorology at the Talcott Mountain Science Center in Avon, Connecticut, and holographic photography at the Weizmann Institute of Science in Israel. Once in college, I became a biology teaching assistant and a physics tutor in addition to my regular schedule of science courses. There was rarely a time when I was not involved in some type of science-related activity. More recently, however, I have discovered that there is another world outside the scientific establishment: one that has made me aware of my inner strengths, my capacity to handle responsibility, and my sensitivity towards other people.

It was in the mountains of Wyoming where I learned the true meaning of challenge. As part of a two-week winter camping and survival course taught by the National Outdoor Leadership School (NOLS), I camped out in temperatures of twenty-seven degrees below zero, cross-country skied with a seventy pound pack, and climbed to altitudes that could not sustain vegetation. Survival, not the allurement of the alpine environment, was my only thought. It was not until I had time to reflect upon my adventures that I realized what it meant to persevere. I knew I could apply those characteristics of determination, will, and desire to any future situation.

My participation in an American Youth Hostel (AYH) leadership training course is where I learned the skills of leadership and responsibility. Here, for the first time, I was responsible for the welfare of others as I conducted a group bicycle tour across Ohio. After nine days of pedaling through the farmlands of Pandora, replacing the broken spokes of Fuji bicycles and settling the common arguments among my companion bikers, i.e., when to eat, whose turn it was to clean up, and how to spend group funds, I understood what responsibility entailed. It was more than directing a group towards a destination. It was listening to their problems and helping each one see different viewpoints. It was consoling a forty-five year-old woman when her rear wheel was hopelessly bent, and it was helping a fellow college student whip up a late dinner for an unruly group.

While the NOLS and AYH programs are just two short experiences in my life, what I took from them has enabled me to see how important people are in my future. I know now that I enjoy working with all types of people, that I will not shy away from difficult problems, and that I have the skills and temperament to handle various situations. This knowledge, coupled with my interest in science, has inspired me to seek a career that combines humanism with scientific expertise.

This summer I have accepted a position in the Hartford Hospital Student Fellowship Program where I am involved in pulmonary function testing under the supervision of Dr. Arthur DeGraff. This program has enabled me to witness certain clinical procedures which have confirmed what I always felt inherent in the medical profession: that physicians are not just scientists but have a concern for other people, are able to persevere in difficult situations, and accept responsibility in life and death matters. While there is a great physical difference between the mountains of Wyoming and the corridors of Hartford Hospital, both have given me a new insight into myself and the medical profession. I now hope to study medicine and become the type of physician who is as comfortable with a stethoscope as he is with a patient's complaint.

# Essay #5

I would like to share a number of personal experiences that contributed to my decision to become a physician.

I first became interested in science in high school when an extremely talented teacher introduced me to the study of biology. Although the course was only an introductory one, this teacher went far beyond the standard curriculum. Not only did the class dissect frogs, grasshoppers, and worms, but it also proceeded under his direction to dissect cow eyes, and the brains and hearts of sheep. As the course progressed, the teacher's enthusiasm for his subject made me, in turn, eager to learn more. Thus my introduction to science at the high school level was very positive, and I looked forward to pursuing a science-related career.

Another high school experience was also to prove instrumental in my future career choice. I was involved in a program in which students volunteered at Suffolk Development Center, a state-run mental institution in Melville, New York. Each volunteer was assigned to one patient on a regular basis. My charge, Joey, was a nineteen-year-old boy, who was blind, mentally retarded, and crippled. Quite frankly, the experience at first made me uncomfortable—I had never before been exposed to such severely handicapped people—but my initial feeling subsided as I became more involved with helping Joey perform simple tasks which, for him, were major accomplishments. This experience made me sensitive to the need to provide facilities for those whose health is mentally or physically impaired, and taught me that patience, care, and determination are needed to help such people. It was at this time that I began to focus on a career in medicine.

Because I was aware that the practice of medicine involved not only scientific principles, but a real understanding of the human condition, I sought in college to place my interest in science within a broad humanist perspective. I particularly enjoyed my Classics courses, and as for my science courses, it was Electron Microscopy that made the deepest impression on me. Here I was able to view in fine detail the complexity of cells and tissues. This course also provided me with an opportunity to work independently—preparing tissue, examining it under the microscope, and analyzing the various histological structures.

During my college years, I was able to observe the practical application of scientific knowledge. For example, I spent the month of January of my sophomore year in the Human Genetics Department of the Yale University School of Medicine. I attended medical school genetics classes, as well as various medical conferences. Most important, however, under the direction of Dr. Xandra O. Breakfield, I engaged in an independent research project involving the bloodstream activity of the enzyme dopamine-B-hydroxylase and its possible basis of genetic inheritance. Although the results of the project were inconclusive, the experience proved to be very helpful to me, because it gave me an understanding of how scientific research can be used to study clinical problems.

My understanding of the field of medicine was enhanced during the following summer when, as a student intern, I was able to observe the activities of physicians in various specialties at Booth Memorial Hospital in Flushing, New York. These specialties included General Surgery, Pathology, Pediatrics, Endocrinology, and Radiology. I also spent time in the Emergency Room, the Clinic, and the Intensive Care Unit. This experience enabled me to appreciate the role of the doctor in both a hospital setting and private practice. In addition, my internship gave me an introduction to the advanced technology used in modern hospitals, and it also allowed me to observe firsthand the more intangible components of the practice of the art of medicine: the care, compassion, and dedication that these professionals demonstrated.

Because my experience at Booth was so valuable, I wanted to use the summer of 1983 to add to my knowledge of the medical field. I applied, therefore, to the Sarah Lawrence Program for Pre-Medical Students at Lawrence Hospital in Bronxville, New York, and I have been accepted. This program attempts to provide an overview of the medical experience while focusing on the students' personal interests. I look forward, in particular, to spending time in Emergency Medicine, Endocrinology, and Pathology.

My various experiences in high school and college have shown me that the field of medicine demands intelligence, integrity, compassion, and commitment, and I believe that my personal attributes will enable me to make a positive contribution to the profession.

# Essay #6

Throughout my young life, I have constantly strived to answer the questions presented before me. Some have been easy—"What is the square root of 9,801?" (99). Others have not been quite so simple—"What do you want to be when you grow up? Why?" My first science courses in the 7th grade stimulated my interest in the medical profession. Before long, I had even selected a speciality: neurosurgery.

Although I have almost always had set goals, I have not been afraid to challenge them. From my sophomore year through my high school graduation, I worked as a typist/computer programmer (15-20 hr/wk, five d/wk) in a small music stand business. This job not only allowed me to improve my dexterity, but also to contribute to my family's strained budget; thus I tasted my first responsibility in the real world. Although I briefly considered a career in computers, I soon realized that I would gain little sense of contribution to other people.

During my first two years in college I worked as an attendant (20 hr/wk) at a local video arcade. Constant interaction with customers made my employment there well worthwhile.

The summer following my sophomore year, I found a job as a lab assistant (30 hr/wk, 1½ mos) in the neuroresearch center of the VA Hospital in Palo Alto, CA. At first I worked as a simple lab technician. Before long, however, my supervisor became convinced that I had the potential to do more, and I was taught to inject rats and to perform a simple surgical maneuver—crush a nerve in the leg and sew the surrounding muscles and skin back together. Although I worked in this lab for a relatively short time, the exposure piqued my interest in the field of research, an option I am currently considering quite seriously.

Acting on this new-found interest in research, I took on a job in the psychobiology labs on Berkeley campus (10-15 hrs/wk, 5 d/wk 1st sem; 5 h/wk, 3 d/wk 2nd and 3rd sems, as projects became less demanding). I wrote two reports while receiving academic credit, describing how a component of long-term memory in rats could be affected by certain drugs. In these papers I designed several original statistical analyses and, in a recently published paper of which I was a co-author, we showed for the first time that long-term memory could be used in a manner not previously considered. Here I was able to interact with professionals as I gained a much more in-depth, rewarding exposure to life in the labs.

In addition to volunteering my time in the labs, I have supported myself by typing an organic chemistry textbook (10-20 h/wk, 5 d/wk; full-time during the summers). This job has been particularly rewarding, as the author allowed me to start editing the book from a student's point of view. My goal has been to present organic chemistry to future students in a clearer and more interesting fashion than it was presented to me.

Although I have enjoyed the challenge of medical research and studies, I have gained increasing satisfaction from contributing my services to others. For the past three years, I have participated in our campus "Buddy" orientation program. Perhaps my greatest satisfaction came when one particular "buddy" (who had been out of school for almost eight years) came to me for help. At first, the shock of university life seemed to be pushing her on the verge of a nervous breakdown, but as I continued to volunteer countless hours of both tutoring (something I have always enjoyed doing) and moral support, she finally began to calm down, and now performs at or near the top of her classes. There may be nothing on this earth more rewarding than helping someone else realize his or her potential!

Having repeatedly reaffirmed my career choice as a physician and/or medical researcher, I realized that I had virtually no experience helping actual patients. Consequently, I started working this February in the ever-busy trauma center at San Francisco General. Before long I found myself working every Friday night from 11 p.m. to 4 a.m., helping physicians and nurses complete a variety of tasks (lab-runs, guerney sheet-changes, etc.). More important, however, my primary role has been to provide moral support to and respond to the needs of often-confused and frightened patients. I have even been able to use my Spanish-speaking ability (acquired in part from my Mexican-American background) to help patients that did not know English. Trauma room life has been so exciting that I constantly find myself watching the physicians at work and helping them in any way possible, even by performing CPR on occasion. The satisfaction I have received in making the patients' visits as pleasant as possible, as well as in making the staff's work a little easier, has been inestimable. At four in the morning, I'm almost never ready to leave!

My biggest question now is no longer whether I want to be a doctor, but whether I want to be a specialist, as earlier planned, or a GP, where my services could be more useful, especially in needy Latin American countries. The decision may not be too difficult if my experiences keep going the way they have been!

# Essay #7

The problems of our society, particularly those related to health care delivery, are numerous. Solutions to these problems will arise from individuals who have a broad view of society and the will to contribute their talents to society. I feel that I possess these qualities and can best contribute my talents to society as a physician.

It was as a junior in high school that I began to consider pursuing a career in medicine. I decided to participate in Project SOAR, a summer premedical program at Xavier. As a participant in Project SOAR, I had the opportunity to learn about medicine by speaking to students who had been accepted by medical schools. By exposing me to college-level work and successful premedical students, whose academic backgrounds were similar to my own, SOAR enhanced my confidence in my academic ability and encouraged me to pursue a career in medicine.

During my senior year in high school, I enrolled as a part-time student in the Concurrent Admissions program at Xavier, where I attended six semester hours of credit. My experiences in Project SOAR and in the Concurrent Admissions program influenced my decision to matriculate at Xavier, full-time, as a chemistry major.

Pursuing a career in medicine is a challenge that should be undertaken only by persons who have a genuine interest in health care. I have learned that I would enjoy working as a physician to improve the quality of health care in our society. My experience in the 1984 United Negro College Fund Summer Premedical Institute affirmed my interest in medicine and provided me with information about a variety of exciting medical careers. I will participate in the 1986 Summer Research Fellowship Program at the Cornell University Medical College, where my research assignment will involve nuclear medicine. Clinical exposure is also a component of the program. I look forward to the experience, since it should provide me with a better understanding of the role of research in medicine.

At Xavier I have had the opportunity to gain teaching experience. I instructed a general chemistry class, one day each week, during the fall semester of 1984, and in 1985 I taught high school students who participated in a summer chemistry program. Assisting my students in reaching their academic goals was very rewarding. Teaching was very enjoyable, because it allowed me to work with people in a meaningful way. I feel that I would enjoy practicing medicine, since it would allow me to interact with people in a similar manner.

Presently I am interested in diagnostic imaging and academic medicine. Because I am very interested in social issues, I am also considering pursuing the degree of Master of Public Health, so that I may better serve the health care delivery system.

Physicians, like other citizens, have a vested interest in the well-being of society. They should be involved not only in treating patients, but also in solving the problems of health care delivery, such as providing medical care to the indigent and the elderly. Although my career goals are not definite at this time, I feel that my background is such that I can pursue a career in any area of medicine and make a meaningful contribution to society. Moreover, my ability to work with others strengthens my conviction that medicine is my vocation. For these reasons, I believe that I can best serve society as a physician.

# Essay #8

During college my closest friends and I have spent hours analyzing our personalities and determining what makes us unique. We explored what motivated our becoming good doctors and why it would make us happy, and we examined the underlying currents which influence and motivate our thoughts and actions. For me, the most visible current is communication: being able to articulate my thoughts, being able to make others experience them, being receptive to the ideas of others, and being understanding.

As a poet, I feel that in order to write meaningful poetry, one must have a clear sense of how to communicate effectively. Whenever I begin a poem, I remember the advice of my high school English teacher: "a poem should be wordless, as the flight of birds." By choosing precise words, by paying attention to the sounds of phrases sewn together, and by evoking clear images, a poem is created. It should grip and move the reader immediately just as a person, seeing a perfectly wedged V-line of Canadian geese flying overhead toward the horizon, stops, catches his breath, and reflects on the beauty that has passed. It is through poetry that I try to recapture my feelings during those wordless moments, and I try to pass them on to the reader.

My need to be a communicator extends beyond poetry. Learning foreign languages, peer counseling, student advising, tutoring, and acting are activities in which I have participated. Each activity emphasizes a particular discipline of communication. Learning foreign languages stems from my enjoyment of communicating with people of different cultures in their native languages. By speaking a language common to us both, communication barriers are bridged. A peer counseling center offers students a comfortable place to talk. By attentive listening, the counselor helps the student clarify his thoughts and feelings and explore options to his problems. Student advisors form quick, friendly rapports with the incoming freshmen. Throughout the year, the advisors offer guidance and suggest options and opportunities at college by relating their own experiences. The tutoring process centers on imparting knowledge. The tutor must motivate the student to cope with his difficulties, to overcome them, and to finally enjoy learning the subject. My involvement in acting and directing is a form of personal expression through interpretation. I draw upon my experiences and intuition to present realistic, complex portrayals. Through foreign languages, peer counseling, student advising, tutoring, and theater, I have explored and developed my communicative abilities. It is this aspect of my personality that will be challenged by a medical career. Whenever one studies foreign languages, one learns to be receptive to a foreign culture. With a perceptive and sympathetic ear is how the peer counselor listens. A student advisor is a freshman's first friend, and a tutor becomes a trusted teacher. An actor or a director investigates the endless possibilities of presenting characters and scenes in certain viewpoints. A doctor embodies the essential characteristics of all these people. A receptive student, a patient listener, an approachable friend, an informative conveyor, and a perceptive examiner are the types of communicator a doctor must be at all times. Recognizing this, I have made a concerted effort to extend and to nurture my capacity for expressing my thoughts, making others experience them, and hearing out the thoughts and ideas of others.

# Essay #9

"John, put another log on the fire." Sparks flew into the night sky. Only the front of me was warm. It was always like that, your back was always cold.

"You still want to be a doctor?"

I nodded.

"In this country you have to be the best. It's the hardest anywhere."

"Then I'll be the best."

"You must rely on yourself. I help as much as is possible, but here only the top get scholarship. In Poland it's easier, but here only a few get the whole shot. I think you can do it if you work hard."

"You know how I work when I want something."

"Yes, I know. Just take a day at a time and you'll do ok."

My father sipped his beer. Silence fell as we watched the flames dance on the logs.

As a young boy I would always look forward to camping with my father. Talk would fly over hundreds of topics as we walked through the forest or sat around the fire at night. He would ramble on about everything from his high blood pressure to nuclear reactions in the sun. Most of the time I never really understood all of what he said, yet I became charmed by the ideas, and thrilled when he would tell me something new. I wanted to know everything, but the more that I knew, the more I realized that I didn't know. Occasionally, I found this to be true too late, as unintentional explosions from my lab in the garage resulted in severe reprimands from my parents.

With age came moderation and a more formal road to education. The innocence of childhood tinkering had matured into the seriousness of adult tinkering, and with it the expectations I had of myself. Although my meager laboratory of childhood was no more, my love for the unknown was alive and well. In the real world though, things seldom went as smoothly as they had in the past.

"I can't get this experiment to work!" I would assert to myself while sitting at my lab bench. "Two o'clock in the morning and two weeks gone by. I swear I'll see these petri-dishes in my sleep. Dr. Youderian always said, 'This is what it's all about.' Indeed, perhaps this time. . ."

Those experiences when things didn't work were just as invaluable as those experiences when things did. After getting to know and appreciate the work and dedication required to discern even the smallest amount of information, it became clear to me why learning in the health sciences is truly lifelong.

Then there were those things which I found one learned only by doing. As a volunteer, I remember one night a young man my age came in with a knife wound to the chest.

"The lung is collapsed," the physician said. There was no time to anesthetize. Five people and myself held the patient down. As the physician made the incision, the boy writhed in pain. The screams made the hair on your neck stand up. As the blood spilled out onto the floor, you could see others around grimace and turn away.

"Look at that guy," I said to my friend nearby in a motion that indicated I was talking about the doctor. "Cool as a cucumber. Just another night at California Hospital for him."

I realized then that there was a lot more to medicine than getting an "A" in a class. I also realized that I still had a long way to go.

For now, that journey is really only beginning. I've taken "a day at a time," and as my father said years ago, I've done "ok." I've worked and planned for a long time, and it's gratifying, as well as slightly frightening, to see it all culminating so quickly now. During those years I hope I've grown and learned such that I might begin a career in medicine. I don't think I ever have been, or ever will be, the "best," but I do know that I've never stopped trying.

# Essay #10

My career goal incorporates biomedical research, treating patients, and teaching. One person who has had particular influence upon this decision is Dr. Michelle Ehrlich. She is a pediatric neurologist who does extensive laboratory research in addition to treating patients. She is extremely effective in both parts of her career, and yet maintains activities outside her profession. Her ability to be a caring physician as well as a successful scientist has reinforced my desire to enter an M.D./Ph.D. program, where I feel I can best acquire the skills necessary for academic medicine.

Scientific research has always intrigued me, as have activities analogous to research, such as games and puzzles that require piecing together acquired items or facts. I enjoy reading the publications of the scientists I have been working with, observing how their results and conclusions evolve, and discussing where their research is heading. I experienced some of this often unpredictable research process myself last semester, while working in the Pharmacology department of the Cornell Veterinary College. In order to learn the techniques used in the lab, I investigated the effects of cobalt and cadmium ions on various properties of mast cells. Although the expected results were reasonably foreseeable, the actual results were not. What began as a laboratory exercise has ended up the topic of my senior honors thesis.

My enthusiasm for research extends beyond strictly basic science into the medical field. I have been working in basic science laboratories in clinical settings, both medical and veterinary. These experiences have stimulated my interest in the clinical applications of basic science research. As an academic physician, I would like to take my own research this one extra step, and have an influence upon the applications of my work. This would further enable me to interact with the patients I would be helping. Additionally, having been hospitalized several times myself, I know the value of a compassionate physician who will spend the extra few minutes explaining the patient's condition and what he or she can expect. Physicians and their patients often have very different ideas of what proper medical care entails, due to different values and beliefs, and it is vital that these differences be considered before any treatment is administered. Frequent patient communication would also help direct my research efforts by allowing me to detect any particular inadequacies in a given treatment and concentrate my work accordingly.

This type of interaction is important in teaching as well. As a teaching assistant for an introductory biology course, I enjoyed explaining ideas that fascinate me and found it particulary gratifying when a struggling student understood a concept with my help. I also liked challenging the more knowledgeable students during quizzes and discussions. They often came up with alternative explanations I had not thought of, teaching me as much as I taught them.

Eventually, I hope to practice medicine in an academic setting, in a position that combines research, teaching, and clinical practice. I feel that the combination of medical and graduate training offered by an M.D./Ph.D. program will enable me to attain this goal.

# Essay #11

I spent my junior year of college at Queens' College, Cambridge University in England. There I studied chemistry and biochemistry (i.e. natural sciences). Credit for my coursework in England is to be applied toward my Cornell University B.A. degree. As of July 14, 1987, the final credit that I will receive for this work does not appear on my official transcript. Also, since I was abroad, I was not able to discuss with my faculty advisor which courses I should take during my senior year. Therefore, my academic record in this application is incomplete. I will notify AMCAS of corrections as soon as possible.

Summer activities:

1985—Volunteer at Pascack Valley Hospital Department of Radiology (Westwood, NJ). Helped with patients, aided x-ray and computer tomography technicians, ran errands for department supervisors.

1986—Lab technician at Rockefeller University (New York City). Conducted synthesis and purification of a protein tumor growth factor (co-researcher of paper pending publication).

1987—Continued research at Rockefeller University. Synthesized and examined analogs of tumor growth factor to discern relationship between structure and activity.

# Essay #12

While exploring a wide range of activities, I discovered an increasing interest in the medical profession. Although desiring a general background, I felt drawn to this field by the challenge and opportunity to employ a variety of my skills and interests in benefitting others in an area of critical need. My love of animals and desire to help the rural worker originally drew me to veterinary medicine and the animal science major. However, after a year of college and exposure to rural areas lacking proper health care, I realized that a greater need existed for physicians.

Exposed to medicine early in life through my mother, a lab technician, and a brother, a doctor, I developed a natural curiosity that led from visits to my mother's lab to volunteering and later working in Clinical Pathology at Upstate. I rotated through the labs performing routine lab tests and became one of the few workers proficient in troubleshooting the equipment. To increase my contact with patients, I requested work as a morning blood-drawer and volunteered in the E.R. The time spent listening to and comforting the patients, especially the elderly, was invaluable.

At college, after performing RIA's for a year in an endocrinology research lab, I resolved to develop a safer assay. The next year was spent researching the alternate methods and finding professors interested in supporting my project. The ELISA method for progesterone in dogs I developed as an undergraduate research project then expanded into my honor's thesis.

Wanting to develop my other interests as well as pursue my goal to become a rural physician, I chose to continue with animal science, a flexible program offerring many of the medically oriented courses. I developed a program strong in genetics and statistics while taking electives in the humanities and computers.

Through travel, reading, work, and various organizations, I pursued my other interests. My work as a computer teaching assistant and terminal operator this year will supplement my programming minor. To act on issues important to me, I joined AgPac, the Curriculum committee, and the campaign committees. Interested in international affairs, I was fortunate to be an Orientation Counselor to the entire International Living Center for foreign students. Enjoying the role of an O.C., I became a student advisor to 12 students, a position with similar but more lasting and personal responsibilities. To further improve my teaching skills, I offerred my services as a tutor through Ho-Nun-De-Kah and worked as a genetics teaching assistant responsible for a 30 student lab section. Riding since high school, I competed throughout the Northeast on the Cornell Riding Team and qualified for Regionals. My continuing interest in horses expanded into organizing horse shows, organizing public service symposiums, and teaching the handicapped to ride. My painting, drawing, and violin playing found an outlet through the various club activities.

These interests remained secondary to and contributed to a growing interest in the social problems facing rural areas. A summer working and living with a farm family and the many conversations we had concerning the difficulties of rural life, confirmed my desire to assist the rural community. At present I work for the Fresh Air Fund Camp which introduces intercity NYC poor and handicapped children to a healthy rural atmosphere while promoting respect for the farmer's role.

Farmers work 80 hour weeks in a high risk job without the benefit of retirement plans, medical plans, paid vacations, or paid sick days. Due to a low population density and thus political invisibility, rural areas frequently suffer from inadequate health care as they are unable to receive even the government support the urban poor receive. In addition, the long hours, understaffing, lack of modern facilities, and isolation in rural practices discourage many physicians.

Aware of these difficulties, I am committed to operating a clinic as a family practitioner, utilizing an effective support staff similar in organization to the Frontier Nursing Service. This practice allows the physicians to use their time more effectively in giving quality and humanistic care. It is my hope to establish such a clinic in a rural area presently lacking in health care.

# Essay #13

Adversity was my transition to maturity. Freshman year was marked by an academic citation, election to dorm council and close friends, but it was also a time of misfortune. I was suspended for three weeks for disorderly conduct due to excessive drinking. As a former dorm proctor, church altar boy and Eagle Scout, I had virtually no experience with drinking. When I returned, I trained as an Alcohol Peer Counselor, and later realized that Dartmouth's party atmosphere was inappropriate for me.

I applied to Northwestern and Cornell. Northwestern immediately accepted me; Cornell accepted me for January admission. After a successful term at Northwestern, I was pleased to join my brother at Cornell and receive a generous scholarship. In addition, Cornell selected me a Transfer Fellow due to my academic and extracurricular record.

Some students with a distruped start as a freshman might give up any aspiration of becoming a doctor. The goal, however, was too important to me. I first considered becoming a doctor ten years ago. I participated in a gifted program at a nearby university. In a biology course, we dissected various organs, wore surgical gloves, and worked with scalpels. I loved it.

During this same time my grandfather, who lived with us, was told he had terminal cancer. He changed from a strong, healthy man to an emaciated skeleton. I recall the helplessness I felt as I watched him slowly die. At twelve, I decided to become a physician.

I examined my ambition more seriously in high school. I founded the Hotchkiss Medical Club. We met many doctors and went on trips to Bridgeport Hospital and Yale University. Everything about medicine fascinated me.

At seventeen I confronted a medical emergency. Mother and I were driving into a shopping center. The driver in the car ahead suddenly slumped over the wheel. I pulled the old, bearded man out of the car and administered CPR. When the ambulance crew arrived, I continued while they did other things to revive the patient. Since then, as a lifeguard at a busy state park, I saved lives; and, as a Red Cross volunteer, I assisted in emergency rooms.

As a senior, I look back on my freshman experience with a

new understanding. People make mistakes. What you do with your life after a setback shows your true worth. As an Alcohol Peer Counselor, I educated others about the perils of excessive drinking. At Northwestern and Cornell, I helped establish similar programs. As a Residential Advisor, Peer Educator, and counselor, I helped freshmen avoid dumb mistakes. In turn, I learned to assist peers with problems of depression, rape, drug abuse, unwanted pregnancy and homosexuality. As an Administrative Orientation Counselor, I trained counselors in listening, leadership, and human relations. Recently, I was selected to the University Hearing Board because of my record of leadership, ethical standards, and genuine concern for others. All of my experiences, both positive and negative, prepared me for the maturity, responsibility, and sensitivity demanded of a physician.

# Essay #14

To work with people, to help them when they are sick, and to find ways to prevent illnesses is a challenge. When I volunteered at the Virginia Home for the Disabled in Richmond, I often felt that many illnesses were preventable. I also had the opportunity to help my father treat patients, and I was always thrilled by the successful administration of medicine.

Academic preparation for medical school initially dominated my school career at the University of Richmond. However, in the last year I, under the tutelage of a professor at the University of Richmond, found myself very involved in a research program which resulted in the publication of a paper. This program taught me how to maintain endurance and interest in an academic area and was therefore the most educational experience in my college career. My communicative and persuasive skills were also developed, for the research involved the competitive procurement of grants as well as the lecturing to audiences of varying backgrounds on the subject matter.

As a result of the emphasis on the research project, I did not take all of the courses required for premedical preparation, but I had an unexpected opportunity to compensate the following year. My original plan was to join the Peace Corps between college and medical school. I succeeded in graduating (cum laude) early. Unfortunately the assignment was delayed for more than a year. It was during this time that I continued to carry on my interest in research. I worked as a laboratory technician and as an assistant in an OB-GYN practice. As a technician in a private laboratory in Massachusetts, I was able to perform supervised experiments in order to identify and isolate clotting factors in Horseshoe crab blood—with possible implications of medicinal value.

Upon moving to Virginia, I began a part-time occupation in an OB-GYN practice. Working in a medical practice has made me realize that the need for communicating information is just as vital as learning it. Therefore, I have tried to prepare myself in this area as well. Being raised in a bilingual (American/German) household, I am at ease in speaking either language. I added Spanish during my first year in college at St. Louis University in Madrid, Spain. Further, being somewhat of a history buff has allowed me to extend my communicative skills as well:

I am currently an active docent for the Fairfax County Park Authority, and thus I give tours at a representative Virginia plantation named Sully.

To some extent travel allowed me insight into the culture, religion, and needs of other people. In addition, another very enlightening experience occurred during the summer of 1983 in Woods Hole, Massachusetts. I partook in a marine research program given by Boston University and was confronted with a vast new area of information in both historic and scientific respects. The summer courses centered on detailed studies and independent research projects dealing with the oceans and their inhabitants. Emphasis was also placed on the individual's ability to cooperate and to withstand the physical hardships that a small crowded sailing vessel foisted upon one. My research project on this cruise resulted in a paper on the polychaete population in the Bay of Fundy.

My recreational hobbies include a wide variety of non-medically oriented activities. For example, I am learning how to play the classical guitar. I maintain a productive herb and flower graden. I enjoy windsurfing in the local waters. During the winter months, I also spend a great deal of time involved in ice skating, skiing, wood carving, and needlecraft. Furthermore, I sew most of my wardrobe. I have been involved with jewelry making, with mechanical car repairs, and with the German School Choir. I also learned some veterinary medicine when my entire family took a summer course at Cornell University Adult Education.

My life has been exciting and diversified. Evenso, I have never lost sight of the quest to become a physician.

# Essay #15

$M$y interest in medicine is rooted in various medically related positions I have held in clinical and research settings. In 1982 I was awarded an NIH summer fellowship at Roswell Park Memorial Institute, Buffalo, New York, where I characterized an anti leukemia-lymphoma monoclonal antibody. This work won the institute's Sydney Farber Award for Outstanding Independent Research. Conducting research in a laboratory associated with several hospitals offered insights into the relationship between basic science and health care. The following summer I worked as a dissector for the Department of Anatomy, State University of New York at Buffalo Medical School, preparing prosections for the gross anatomy course. I enjoyed both the analytical approach of laboratory research and the precision of dissection: hence I sought further experience in the biomedical field.

During my freshman year at Cornell I applied to the College Scholar Program as a means of combining interests in the biological and social sciences. Under the auspices of this program, competitively selected undergraduates design their own majors, integrating broad topics not accommodated by the usual curriculum. I am pursuing concentrations in cell biology and Soviet studies.

In the summer of 1984 I worked as an emergency room volunteer at the Buffalo General Hospital. At the same time, as a Summer Research Fellow at the Department of Oral Biology, State University of New York at Buffalo Dental School, I prepared monoclonal antibodies against the oral pathogen *Actinobacillus actinomycetemcomitans*. These antibodies have since been patented by the university. This intensive, simultaneous exposure to biomedical reseach and clinical practice firmly established my resolve to pursue a career in medicine. It also persuaded me of the importance of research as a foundation underlying medical practice; consequently I have used the flexibility of the College Scholar Program to integrate research into my academic work. I substituted an independent research project of characterizing an *Apium graviolens* enzyme, in the course of which I used most basic biochemical techniques, for the traditional biochemistry lab course. Upon completion of this project I began research on the structure and function of glucose-6-phosphatase in conjunction with work being performed in the laboratory of Dr. William Arion, Department of Biochemistry, Molecular and Cell Biology, Cornell University.

Currently I am participating in the DeBakey Summer Program at the Department of Surgery, Baylor College of Medicine. I assist in cardiovascular surgery under Dr. E. Stanley Crawford at the Methodist Hospital of Houston, and work during my free time at the emergency room and trauma center of the nearby Benjamin Taub county hospital. Through this experience I have learned, by direct participation, aspects of the day-to-day reality of cardiovascular surgery and trauma care; happily found myself capable of maintaining a first year intern's hours; and, by working with patients in two so vastly different institutions, have been stimulated to reconsider some social aspects of the health care delivery system.

# Essay #16

$M$y interest in becoming a physician has developed through exposure to both clinical medicine and investigative research. In the first area, I have had the opportunity to work in the office practice of an ophthalmologist and to observe surgery at three hospitals. In college, I successfully completed an Emergency Medical Technician training course. Throughout these experiences, I was impressed and inspired by the skill, dedication and compassion of the professionals with whom I worked and studied.

I was introduced to investigative medicine during an eight-week paid fellowship in the Tissue Typing Laboratory of the New York Blood Center. In this position I learned the basic histocompatability tests necessary to match donors with recipients for kidney and bone marrow transplantation and studied the relationship between specific HLA factors and certain diseases such as Juvenile Macular Degeneration.

With a strong recommendation from the Blood Center, I procured a salaried position of greater scientific complexity and responsibility at Memorial Cancer Center in the Summer of 1984. My extensive work in the immunohematology laboratory of Memorial has been the single most significant force in my decision to attend medical school.

The first summer I was responsible for establishment and maintainance of several of the first cell lines derived from patients with Acquired Immunodeficiency Syndrome (AIDS) and the analysis of AIDS patients' immune response through measurement of lymphocyte transformation and Natural Killer Cell activity *in vitro*. I was the only student approved to work in the P-3, biological containment level, laboratory that year.

In 1984, there was very little documentation concerning the transmission and prognosis of AIDS. Our research was directed at determining the efficacy of several drugs in restoring AIDS patients' immune response. Although I was working with patient blood in a high-containment facility and had realistic concerns for the safety of myself and others working in the laboratory, I felt extremely fortunate to have the opportunity to use my recently acquired skills and to learn new procedures within a formal research design. My greatest satisfaction was observing the connection between what we were accomplishing in the laboratory and the plight of the AIDS patients with whom I met and talked.

During the following January, I returned to the immunohematology laboratory at Memorial where I was given the opportunity to continue with my work at a more sophisticated level and with more independence. My research during this month was aimed at determining whether the antigenic agent recognized when normal Natural Killer cells lyse AIDS target cells is similar to the antigen expressed by Epstein-Barr virus-infected cells.

This past summer I returned again to the laboratory to assist in supervising and was assigned to train new members of the team, one of whom was a doctor doing a fellowship in our laboratory. This was the summer of the greatest recognition of the importance of the AIDS virus and anxiety about transmission into the population outside the previously accepted high-risk groups. Strengthening the containment levels and adding additional precautions, I tested a newly proposed drug for AIDS, investigated the cell-mediated immunity of growth hormone-deficient patients, continued to maintain cell lines and learned a new interferon assay.

While I plan to defer my decision as to which field I will specialize in until after completion of my basic science studies, my experience at Memorial over the last two years has convinced me of my aptitude and interest in investigative research. However, in whatever field I choose, I will not divorce myself from patient care, for it was the personal interaction with patients that made my laboratory experience most meaningful.

# Essay #17

My interests in biomedical science and the performing arts developed while I was a youngster. Fortunately, I have been able to enjoy both fields.

Since May 1985, I have been working part-time during classes and full-time during breaks as a research technician at NIH, in Dr. John E. Folk's group (Natl. Inst. of Dental Research, Laboratory of Oral Biology and Physiology, Enzyme Chemistry Section). I assist Dr. Myung Hee Park. The focus of our work is one of the eukaryotic protein synthesis initiation factors, eIF-4D, a protein which contains the unusual amino acid hypusine (N -(4-amino-2-hydroxybutyl)lysine) as the result of post-translational modification: a lysine residue receives the butylamine portion of spermidine and is subsequently hydroxylated. The functions of the factor and its hypusine residue are unknown at this time. In Sept. 1985, I was assigned my own project, the molecular cloning and sequencing of cDNA coding for eIF-4D. A bacteriophage lambda gt11 human hepatoma expression library was screened with oligonucleotide and antibody probes, and DNA sequencing experiments are currently underway. During the summer of 1985, I was engaged in the purification of eIF-4D from human erythrocytes by multistep chromatography and differential precipitation, analyzing the product by SDS-PAGE, LPLC and amino acid analysis. I am a coauthor of two papers and one abstract which describe that summer's work.

At George Mason University, I worked from Dec. 1983 to Sept. 1984 as research assistant to Prof. Suzanne Slayden of the Chemistry Department, studying the competition between protonolysis and rearrangement in certain trialkylboranes. In addition to learning the required air-sensitive techniques, I routinely analyzed the products using GC and proton NMR. From Aug. 1984 to the present, I have been working with Dr. Slayden on a series of instructional videotapes designed to introduce various forms of spectroscopy to students of organic chemistry. These programs feature computer graphics and animations which I created in my spare time. One of them—"Interpreting NMR Spectra"—will be presented at the American Chemical Society's Mid-Atlantic Regional Meeting in Baltimore.

Prior to my return to college, I worked from Jan. 1980 to July

1983 as a Senior Research Technician at The New York Blood Center, assisting Dr. Bernard Horowitz of the Blood Derivatives Program. Dr. Horowitz provided me with a working tutorial in experimental and process-scale protein chemistry, and eventually encouraged me to complete my formal education. My first year in his lab produced a chromatographic method for the purification of human leukocyte interferons. I characterized the material using isoelectric focusing, SDS-PAGE and 2D-PAGE, comparing the distribution of interferon subtypes in the highly-purified chromatographic eluate to those in the non-recombinant interferon preparations then approved for use in human clinical trials. My efforts were then directed to the purification and characterization of human Factor VIII:C. Its association with von Willebrand factor was probed, and a number of RIAs and ELISAs were developed. The final phase of my work with Dr. Horowitz grew out of the AIDS epidemic: I investigated several methods of chemically inactivating viruses in blood products, aiming for conditions which were benign to Factor VIII procoagulant activity, yet left the injectables virus- and reagent-free. This project was passed on to other workers when I returned to school. I was a coauthor of two abstracts describing some of the interferon and Factor VIII work.

My laboratory experience also includes eighteen months (1978-80) as a clinical laboratory technician at Pathology Associates Laboratories in Beverly Hills, CA. I was responsible for running the daily "panel" of blood chemistries on an automated analyzer and flame photometer, and routinely performed RIAs and inoculated cultures. Other ongoing duties included the preparation of samples and the logging of patient information. I was intially hired as a courier by this lab, but was promoted into the laboratory at my request.

From 1971 to 1978, I was a performer (actor, singer and guitarist). I appeared in three Broadway shows, four national tours and numerous radio and television broadcasts. My association with the pathology lab started as one of the many jobs between shows, but proved to be the beginning of a new and more satisfying career, one free of the cyclic unemployment of the actor's life. My training in drama and music has proven to be a valuable asset in the biomedical field: an actor is taught to prepare and empathize; a musician develops manual dexterity and structured study habits; both must adapt to a wide variety of environments, and both require the ability to work in tandem with people of diverse backgrounds and interests.

# Essay #18

I have wanted to become a doctor since I first watched my ophthalmologist father treat patients and since I learned that I was born with a tracheo-esophogeal fistula, and first wondered at the miracle of modern medicine that had occurred inside my own body. Yet, these realities have very little to do with my desire to become a physician today: over the past several years, an intuition has been transformed into an informed, intellectual motivation.

I spent two summers during high school as a volunteer counselor at ANCHOR, a camp for emotionally, physically, and mentally handicapped children and adults in New York. The work was demanding (I spent hours each day lifting arms and legs during exercise classes, helping women change into swimsuits for the beach, running after missing campers) and emotionally challenging (many of the men and women were verbally abusive and physically threatening—more of them were depressed) but, by the end of my first summer, a camper whom I had been guiding had gained enough confidence to step into the pool on a hot day: this was all the reward I needed.

Eager to explore the psychological and psychiatric problems that I have encountered recreationally, in the summer after my Freshman year, I worked at Payne Whitney Hospital as a research assistant on an NIMH study of the effectiveness of family therapy intervention for inpatients with schizophrenia and major affective disorders. I tabulated data, contacted subjects, performed follow-up interviews, observed group therapy, attended team conferences and made rounds with the residents and senior staff. I experienced some of the challenges of research: I saw instances where the protocol came into conflict with a patient's best interest; I realized how challenging it could be to get subjects to maintain their commitment to the project. I observed many of the frustrations and rewards of clinical psychiatry: in the last week of the summer one patient tried to commit suicide for the fourth time and another went home to her family and her job.

The following summer, I worked on a NIH study of juvenile macular degeneration at Manhattan Eye, Ear, Nose and Throat Hospital. I had designed a statistical form for diagnosis retrieval and was assisting in the epidemiological study when the staff nurses and ancillary personnel at the hospital walked out on a strike. Since I had recently completed an emergency medical technician training course, I volunteered to substitute for striking workers in the emergency department. The emergency room held wonders that I had not imagined from the seclusion of the retinal research laboratory upstairs: I tested the visual acuity of elderly women with glaucoma and of people who spoke only Spanish or Polish or Greek; I listened to the fears of a concerned parent of an infant with a corneal ulcer; I comforted a young girl who was having a cockroach removed from her ear; I explained the importance of self-assessment vision testing to a man with macular degeneration. When a woman walked in one night with an orbital fracture and a facial laceration, I held her hand as the plastic surgeon placed fifteen stitches in her cheek. I stopped a woman as she tried to snap a leather belt in front of the eyes of her pre-school child: the resident had just treated him for a corneal abrasion. Through the otoscope and the slit-lamp biomicroscope—on my first day—I saw a ruptured ear drum and a herpes dendritic corneal ulcer. From week to week as patients returned for follow-up examinations, I tested their visual acuity and excitedly watched the return of their vision.

Also at MEETH, I witnessed the struggles of people who could not afford to purchase medical care. I spoke with a man who had allowed his pterygium to progress beyond the point of reversible sight loss: he told me that he had waited to come in because he knew he would not be able to pay. Throughout the summer, many of the complexities of health care provision for a diverse group of patients became evident to me: I lost an image of my father treating macula patients in his office and gained a more complicated and, for me, more fascinating portrait of medical care. To assimilate my new ideas, I enrolled at the London School of Economics for a year's study of social policy and health administration.

In London and at the LSE, I studied and searched for answers to some of the questions I had posed while working in the emergency room. At Williams I had trained to be a contraception and health counselor to my peers: at the LES, I studied family planning policies in the United States, the United Kingdom, and China. As I sat in the offices of my health care administration professors—all of whom had advisory positions within the National Health Service—I rediscovered a personal talent that had been overshadowed by years of English and pre-medical courses. At Horace Mann High School, I had distinguished myself in organization and leadership as the elected Chairman of both the Allocations Committee and the Governing Council. At Williams, I had been selected by the college president to serve as one of three student representatives on the board of Trustees' Committee on Priorities and Resources. At the LSE, I learned that what had enabled me to work effectively on these committees was essential to the role of health policy, breastfeeding in the Third World, provision of emergency care in the NHS and the relationship between race and health and I wrote papers and delivered class lectures with an interest that was unparalleled in all of my past academic work.

Yet, for all the gratification and intellectual excitement I found studying health care administration, I never discarded my intention to become a doctor: rather, my experience has more firmly convinced me of the correctness of my choice. Now, I am prepared and anxious to study medicine with a full awareness that medical decisions and problems have social and political roots and implications and a full consciousness of the essential humanity of medical practice.

# Essay #19

I have never understood the great hullabaloo some people raise about a conflict between science and the humanities. All my life I have been attracted to both and am puzzled by the perspective of a friend who claims, "I'm not a 'science person,'" or some of my fraternity brothers who raise their brows when I register for a class in poetry writing. As a profession, I feel medicine will allow me to live in both worlds.

I enjoy learning about lots of different things, so school has always been easy and fun. I also take great pride in being competent in many areas, from basketball and windsurfing to tutoring math and cooking chicken paprikash. For as long as I can remember, I have been an addict of the animal shows appearing on television. I love watching polar bears plunging through ice and close-ups of frogs laying jelly-covered eggs. But I never aspired to be shooting those films, knee deep in mire or perched in a tree, and I don't want to be a veterinarian. When I first entered high school I wanted to direct films, modeling myself after Francois Truffaut. Later I decided I would satisfy this desire with artful home movies or perhaps by assisting in a medical documentary. Writing fiction is one of my favorite hobbies and I would love, some day, to try publishing a novel.

Of all my interests, I have a special passion for biology which I expect everyone to share. The magic in living things which transcends molecular and cellular analysis makes studying them the most interesting thing I can imagine. So when someone blurts, "Ugh! I hated biology in high school!" I smile but honestly wonder if he is crazy. My research experience of two summers in a neuroimmunology lab at Columbia intensified this conviction and made me even more excited about my plans to study medicine.

There is a tradition of doctors on both the Cuban and Hungarian sides of my family, but it was only late in high school that I decided for sure that I wanted to study medicine myself. When my older brtother, now studying at Mount Sinai, decided to go into medicine, I chose all my high school courses in areas outside natural science. Gradually, I realized that I could still like science, or consider a medical career, without just copying my brother. Volunteering in the emergency room at Columbia Presbyterian last summer was the final step I needed to evaluate my commitment to medicine and it has made me sure that I am doing the right thing. I sought out the smelliest and bloodiest patients, changing their bed pans and bringing them water, and once helped restrain a woman having heart seizures while blood streamed from a catheter in her nose. I found that actively helping made these experiences less and less gross and unexpectedly emboldened me to tackle something bigger. I was also inspired by the exciting side of medicine, rushing to the trauma room in any free moment to watch the surgeons clean and stitch wounds. Sometimes I caught myself grinning on the subway ride home, wondering if some day I would be sewing wounds myself.

Though I welcome excitement and intellectual satisfaction, what I really want from my career is to feel I am channeling a lifetime of energy into something meaningful and worthwhile. As compared to a career in business, or directing films, I believe studying and practicing medicine will fulfill this need. The greatest asset I have to offer is my motivation, to give and to work, to become as good a doctor as I am able to. Beside a warm family and close friends, there is truly nothing I want more and nothing that would make me happier.

# Essay #20

The rate at which medical knowledge is moving along today has brought out the necessity for two very important qualities in physicians: an open mind, which will recognize the advantages and, at the same time, limitations of new technologies and practising methods, and a high degree of adaptability, which will allow these new methods to be effectively integrated into medical practice.

I believe that my life experience reflects such qualities. Throughout my education I have tried to keep an open mind and expand my horizons. Making the decision to come to the United States for my college education was a step in that direction. Prior to that, I had spent significant periods of time in Africa (Zambia, Ghana and Morocco), and in travelling through Europe. My stay in Morocco was particularly interesting: I witnessed the efforts of an ambitious ruler to inspire a fascinating but at times distorting process of modernization along western models.

I spent the latter part of my schooling at Campion School in Athens, Greece, which prepares students according to the British educational system. Although my high school community was small and rather close-knit, its environment was limiting only to those who chose to find limits in themselves. Besides my placing first in my graduating class, I was active in student government, classical drama, three varsity sports, and classical guitar performances. At the same time I came to develop a keen interest in the biological sciences and a fascination for the humanitarian aspects of medicine.

Coming to the University of Pennsylvania to explore the field of Biology was a major decision which I took conscious of the new directions it would open up for me. The environment was quite different from any other I had known before, but I needed the challenge to see how valuable my previous experiences really were. After all, my intention had always been to build for myself a perspective which would give me a good degree of awareness and adaptability. Admission to the highly competitive University Scholars program and my success in gaining a place on the varsity soccer team placed me in a very challenging milieu within the university. I believe I responded well. Academically, my program of liberal arts studies reached deep into the process of intellectual enrichment which I consider to be basic to the notion of scholarship. In sports, I became the top varsity goal scorer in the 1984-1985 season and was voted most improved player.

My motivation is a tool which I love to put to use in causes that I feel are worthwhile. This is reflected in the significant broadening of activities at the Penn Greek Club since December, 1985, when I took office as President. We began to organize a series of lectures and films on issues as diverse as recent political developments in Greece, the restoration of Athenian monuments, and the Olympic theme. The response was quite rewarding: our club membership eventually tripled.

I have come to regard medicine as a field where the practitioner is in a constant, intimate relationship with science while drawing on much more than just pure science. This dialectic process holds a special appeal for me. In my mind, emphasis in medical care should be as much on "care" as on the "medical" or scientific aspect. Furthermore, I recognize medicine as a field flexible enough for one to follow his own particular course, and even open up new ways. I see, for example, that in the future the dedicated physician may need to become more and more associated to the statesman and the law-maker; the effects that medical advances have in shaping society and culture are too great for medicine to be regarded solely as an intellectual enterprise. This of course entails expanded responsibilities. I feel capable of contributing to the undertaking.

# Essay #21

During the past year, as I was finalizing decisions about my career choice I have had to accept a more realistic picture of the medical profession than one I had in the past. Based on talks I have had with some physicians, I have gained a better understanding of some of the current problems in medicine. I have also gained a better appreciation of the dedication and devotion of these physicians. These conversations, which at first shocked me, eventually fueled a growing interest that I had in medicine.

Though a medical career had been a consideration since high school, it remained one of several considerations until I began to concentrate in the sciences and accumulate some experience in the area during college.

During the summer of my sophomore year at Cornell, I worked in a reagents research and development lab for a supplier of hospital diagnostic equipment. After deriving improved reagents for spectrophotometric blood analyzers, I tested the accuracy of the new formulas. My summer at Instrumentation Labs proved helpful in future work because I had a chance to familiarize myself with a more sophisticated lab.

In the spring of my junior year I worked with Dr. W.R. Butler of the Physiology Department at Cornell, researching endogenous opiates in rats. In addition to localizing a source of the opiates in the adrenal medulla, I was able to achieve an acetylcholine dependant surge in opiate secretion from the adrenal. Dr. Butler guided me in establishing a credible experimental design, and technicians have introduced me to a number of relevant assay techniques. In the fall, I will be investigating the possible role of opiates integrated with pituitary and/or hypothalamic hormones in regulating the stress response of rats.

This past summer I worked in the Thyroid Diagnostic Center of the Brigham and Women's Hospital for Dr. P.R. Larsen, director of the unit, and Dr. Ira Mills, a Ph.D. doing postdoctoral work in endocrinology. I studied deiodination of thyroid hormone (mainly in the form of T4) to triiodothyronine (T3). T3 has been shown to be a much more active form of the hormone, but T4 is the more predominant thyroid product, thus the conversion is important physiologically. An enzyme similar to the one responsible for the deiodination leading to most of the circulating T3 has been found in brown adipose tissue and may be involved in non-shivering thermogenesis. I investigated the effects of various hormonal treatments on this enzymatically mediated conversion and described receptor mechanisms operating in isolated cells. I have learned conventional biochemical lab procedures, such as RIA's and electrophoresis techniques, and have also had the chance to absorb some of the expertise of the physicians and Ph.D's with whom I have worked. Additionally, while at Brigham and Women's, I have attended lectures given by hospital and lab personnel.

This recent experience has served to focus my career interests. While in school I have enjoyed studying endocrinology and immunology, and I would like to go on to study internal medicine. Eventually, I want to work in a university affiliated hospital, and to be involved in clinically related research, while maintaining patient contact.

At Cornell I have probed some of my other interests, including economics, psychology and politics, as well as taken rigorous science courses which have prepared me well for the demanding curriculum at medical school. I have been an ambassador for the Arts and Sciences School for the past two years during which I have housed prospective Cornellians and have given tours to their families. Also, as a Biology Student Advisor, I have been responsible for advising a group of ten freshmen each year about the biology program at Cornell. In the 1986-87 school year I will be a Resident Advisor in a predominantly freshman dorm. I expect the challenges and rewards to be tremendous.

Medicine interests me because it is often adjusting to new technology and ideas. A career in medicine excites me, not only because of my interests but because it is an opportunity for me to do something I think I could do well while deriving the gratification that comes from helping people.

# Essay #22

I find myself trying to answer the question "Why do you want to be a doctor?" Such a question seems to demand an organized and logical response which I can produce without much trouble, but which is only answers instead of reasons: "I am interested in sciences; I like people; I think it would be exciting." My own answer to myself is more simple, yet more inexplicable—simply that the closer I get to medical practice, the more I like it and the better "gut-feeling" I get about my decision to pursue it. It is our feelings we react to, the justification comes afterwards. Thus I find myself only able to offer a logical rationalization of the emotional responses that are my actual motivation to pursue medicine.

In contrast to many of my fellow pre-meds at Cornell, I entered college with no intention of ever pursuing medicine as a career. I had always been interested in wildlife and environmental studies. I travelled as far as Maine and Alaska in ecological study programs. I taught myself taxidermy and museum preservation skills. In fact it was Cornell's reputation in ornithology that led me to Ithaca. Yet as I became more deeply involved in animal behavior studies, I started to feel a nagging uncertainty as to whether wildlife research was indeed all that I wanted. Realizing that I might be continuing in this study more by inertia than conviction, I decided to take a semester leave of absence to assist a Cornell doctoral student in his research on mockingbird behavior in Texas, hoping to decide whether I really wanted to continue in this direction. After a month or two of this research, I found that the aesthetics of the environment still moved me, but everyday we were working on the same problem, and it quickly became apparent that the results could never justify the effort to me. I grew frustrated with the often myopic intensity of this form of research, and the way an individual's success or failure seemed to depend only on the substance of his thesis, to the apparent exclusion of the content of his character.

Having abandoned what I had always assumed would be my destined career, I used much of my free time in Texas for introspection and soulsearching, trying to decide what I wanted and valued in my life. It was a fascination with science that drew me into biology originally, and though pure research appears too tightly focused to satisfy me, I still enjoy studying science immensely. But I also know that science means more to me if it is linked to individual people. I have decided that medicine or teaching would be the best way for me to stay involved in science, since each incorporates the humanistic qualities that pure research has not seemed to require; and knowing myself, I think that I will be more happy as the doctor rather than the teacher.

My experience this summer has given me added confidence in my decision to pursue medicine. I have been working as a surgical scrub tech in the Johns Hopkins Hospital Gynecology Operating Room. Every day I am scrubbed and in the middle of surgery, sometimes for six hours at a time, handing instruments, threading sutures, retracting, and always asking questions. I have never enjoyed a job more and I truly can't think of anything I would rather be doing this summer, (and certainly nothing else that would get me out of bed at 5:30 a.m. every day). Even when I know nothing about the patient, the science and the surgical technique are fascinating, but when I can talk to the patient and develop at least some personal contact, the science suddenly becomes medicine and it takes on new meaning, for it is that personal contact that moves me the most.

When Helen Avery said good-bye to me for this summer with tears in her eyes, saying she didn't know what she was going to do without me, I realized the feeling that is probably my strongest motivation. She is 87 years old, with two artificial knees, and the beginnings of Parkinson's disease, but she is still the sharpest of all the elderly that I visited last year. Every Friday afternoon I went to see her, sometimes to go for a walk, sometimes to take her shopping, but mostly just to talk. I cannot describe how good it felt to know that my presence mattered, to see her light up and smile when she opened the door for me. As a doctor, hopefully, I can find that feeling again and again. The science may interest me, the diagnoses may challenge me, but it will be that personal involvement with the patient that will make the most difference to me and keep me going through the hardest parts.

# Essay #23

$M$y interest in the field of medicine is the product of a life-long process of discovery which began when I was a child. My mother, a clinical pathologist, and my father, a research pathologist, were responsible for many of the early experiences which sparked my interest in medicine. Through such experiences, I was exposed to many facets of the field, from wonderous triumphs to harsh realities. As a child, I would frequently visit my parents' laboratories. My father would demonstrate the uses of many modern pieces of equipment, often allowing me to look through his electron microscope, while my mother would show me her patients' slides, explaining the reasons for the various and too often malignant diagnoses.

My summer experiences have given me several opportunities to examine the field of medicine first-hand. During the past three summers, I have worked at NYU Medical Center on projects which have provided me with some perspective on both the clinical and basic-science aspects of medicine. At the Rusk Institute, I worked with a team which rehabilitated stroke and accident victims, both physically and emotionally, and I thus became familiar with some of the basic requirements of patient care. In the Department of Hematology, my research for the past two summers focused on the glycoprotein IIb-IIIa complex, which comprises the fibrinogen receptor site on the surface of the platelet membrane. One aspect of this research dealt with investigating the mechanism of Post Transfusion Purpura, a platelet incompatability disorder caused by $PLA_1$, an antigen present on most individuals' glycoprotein IIIa. Consequently, I performed numerous experiments utilizing electrophoresis techniques as well as monoclonal antibodies in Western Blot procedures.

While these projects have served to confirm the intellectual basis for my interest in medicine, non-academic events have shaped my emotional commitment to the field. Through my three-year participation in the Veterans Administration Hospital Volunteers Program, I have derived immense satisfaction by providing conversation and companionship to lonely elderly patients and younger veterans with psychiatric disorders. At the Rusk Institute, I was able to witness and share in the joy patients feel upon slowly regaining strength in their limbs. All of these experiences have made me dramatically aware that physicians have an unparalleled opportunity to help others; this prospect, more than any other, has become my major inducement towards a career as a physician.

# Essay #24

I have been a springboard diver for half of my life. I started at age ten, and by the time I was thirteen I was training six days a week, not because my coach or my parents told me to, but because I loved it. Diving has been my most consistent undertaking over the years; it is the unifying thread that has not only given me immense pleasure, but that has also helped me to grow and to become the person I want to be. As I look back, I see the few material gains diving has given me, such as travel and college offers, but more importantly, I see the vast personal gains it has provided: The ability to do hard work, the ability to honor a committment, the mastery of fear, the experiences of success and self-confidence, and the ability to achieve, to be successful in the face of competition, the ability to sacrifice to achieve the goals I have set.

Diving has given me much, but it has not always been fun. The competition and the mastery of a new dive are what make the sport worthwhile for me, but to achieve these moments of beauty, long hours of practice are necessary—through the winter months, through the times when my friends were out enjoying themselves, through the times when I was not well or was tired. To succeed, I have had to set hard, specific goals for myself, such as becoming a High School All-American (which I achieved), winning the New York State Empire Games (which I did), qualifying for the NCAA Division I Championships (which I have not yet done), and becoming an NCAA All-American (which I most probably will never be). When I think about sleeping and missing a morning workout, or going off with my friends, I recall my goals and realize that I need every bit of practice I can get. Diving has made me realize something that guides me throughout my life: If I want to achieve badly enough, I must make sacrifices now to reach my goals.

As I have progressed, I have gained self-confidence and pride from my ability to work hard for what I want. Also, I have over and over conquered an emotion that feels good to conquer, fear; fear of hitting the board, fear of hitting the water, fear of being out of control 33 feet in the air, fear of performing and exposing my inner self to crowds, fear of failure. I, and all other divers, have experienced all these, many times over. I have really hurt myself, really embarassed myself. What has been most important to me, though, is the ability I have gained to force myself back up there, to try the dive again, to dive in front of the same old crowd the next week. When I can, and can later succeed, the fear goes away, and the confidence in overcoming the fear grows.

Diving has taught me, too, the concept of balance. In college we work out from three to five hours a day, and from December to March have long trips to compete elsewhere. I, like all athletes, have learned how to study when I am tired after workouts. I have learned how to dive and live my life at the same time, how to study and have fun while upholding the athletic standards I have chosen. I have also learned how to maintain my body and my mind, how to elicit the best performance possible, and how to remain healthy when my performance or the team's success depends on it. I have learned to think when I am tired.

I have been successful at the sport, and it has influenced my way of life and my ways of thinking. I believe the qualities that I have gained from diving will help me to be successful in medicine. I have the ability to work hard, experience physical discomfort and mental fatigue, and continue to think and perform well. I can make sacrifices to achieve goals I believe in. I believe that I have the maturity and emotional stability to cope with the rigors of a doctor's education and life, and the personal integrity that will enable me to uphold the trust and responsibility placed in a doctor. And I will always retain my sense of balance—to take all that life can throw at me and turn it to my best advantage. Diving and medicine are both paradoxical— one must strive for perfection, but must realize that perfection will never be reached. To succeed in medicine is my main goal for the rest of my life; it is a goal I believe I can achieve.

# Essay #25

$M$y growing up in a medical family was probably what provided the initial impetus for my interest in a medical career. However, it is my own experiences, apart from my family, which have made it clear to me that this choice is truly based on what I want to do with my life.

My mother is a physician and she has provided a meaningful role model for me. I was aware throughout, of her ability to combine concern for helping people with their medical problems with a strong concern for each individual. I was impressed with her investment in seeing that each patient received the best possible medical care and her ability to combine patient care with ongoing research—research which led to some significant contributions in the area of treatment. My father's position, as I was growing up, as the Medicaid administrator for the city, brought home to me the issues related to equitable delivery of medical care. His devotion of much of his adult life to a program that was a step in the direction of providing medical care for all people in need, regardless of income or insurance regulations, has hopefully made a difference in people's lives.

It is the experiences which I have had, however, which have been important in furthering my understanding of the complexities and realities of the life of a physician. The volunteer work which I did at the Health Sciences Center exposed me to the kind of research which needs to be ongoing in relation to medical problems, and which ultimately contributes to improved patient care. The painstaking work which I was engaged in, in translating CAT scan data onto computers was part of an attempt to clarify how bone conformation relates to locomotion. I can see such data being used in a variety of preventive ways—as for example, in rehabilitation after injuries, in determining the amount of stress an athlete can withstand and in cases of osteroperosis, among others.

My work in the Orthopedic Department at County Medical Center has shown me even more sharply than any previous experience, the complex nature of the skills which contribute to making the competent, caring physician. The in-depth understanding of the human body, the complicated skills needed in performing surgery and the need to find ways of dealing with the tragedies which physicians are confronted with, present a lifelong challenge. To see a 30 year old woman die on the operating table after having jumped in front of a train makes one wonder what was going on in her life that led her to do this. But it is also clear that while the physicians were working to save her, the need was to focus on the medical-surgical tasks confronting them. I could see that the young men who become paraplegic and quadraplegic as a result of motorcycle and water accidents need doctors who can help them with their medical needs and help them go on with their lives. But maybe doctors can also play a role in education for prevention.

I believe at this time that my interest lies in orthopedics. However, I am aware that much lies before me as I hope to start my medical education, and that I need the education, training and exposure to the full range of medicine, before making a lifelong commitment to a specialty.

# Essay #26

My interest in medicine has developed over many years. As a child and adolescent, my parents and relatives filled our home with keen and insightful discussion of the profession. Both of my grandfathers were doctors, two of my uncles are cardiologists, and on one side of the family the tradition goes back four generations—when medicine could hardly claim to be a science. The decision, however, to become a physician has developed in college as an ungentle fusion of my two majors: physics and English. I refrained from a conservative curriculum at the undergraduate level and this combination allowed me a full dose of the humanities and a strong foundation in the physical sciences.

While I continue to enjoy the abstract nature of these disiplines, I consider medicine the practical union of these academic interests: scientific procedures will produce undeniable results, and yet behind each physical ailment will be an individual with special needs and priorities. The double-edged nature of the health profession requires a divided perspective.

My summer work over the last several years further guided my interests in medicine. As a YMCA camp counselor, I gained great satisfaction working closely with others. Moreover, the importance of qualified medical attention and knowledge was driven home to me. As waterfront director, I taught Advanced Lifesaving to all the staff. One summer, one counselor dove into shallow water and injured his neck. A recently trained counselor recognized the cause of his friend's inactive prone position and carefully turned him over allowing him to breathe until the paramedics and doctor arrived to safely immobilize his neck.

Two summers ago, while working on a survey crew on a remote Navajo reservation in Arizona, I was fascinated by the need for culturally sensitive medical care. Good doctors there learned to explain their work and ask questions in ways that demonstrated an understanding of and a respect for a proud culture. Yet the need for primary care physicians was painfully obvious; the bubonic plague made its appearance several times that summer.

This past summer, I was privileged to work in West Germany with two renal physiologists, Dr. Beyenbach of Cornell University and Dr. Fromter of the Max Planck Institute. Earlier that year I had gained general lab experience working in Dr. Beyenback's lab at Cornell. Because of this experience, they allowed me to work quite independently to develop my own skills of physiological investigation.

Our main interest was ion specific channals present in the membranes of collecting duct cells in the mammalian kidney. To study channals, we employed the rather recent technique of patch clamp as developed by the German physiologist Neher. This technique uses tiny glass pipettes to electrically isolate small portions of a cell membrane. Channals can then be detected by the small currents that arise when ions of a specific polarity flow through the small pores of the membrane. I will present the results of this research this December at the American Society of Nephrology's Annual Meeting.

While my work this past summer proved by general abilities in research, I plan to practice medicine at the clinical level. Several factors influence this choice. First of all, I am a person of practical abilities. Although I often enjoy theoretical considerations, I consider myself to be most effective and useful dealing with individual problems. Secondly, I enjoy involvement with a variety of people and a variety of problems. Finally, I favor a more holistic approach in medicine, and toward that end I intend to practice primary-care medicine as a Family Practitioner.

# Essay #27

A successful and effective physician must possess two essential qualities—a thirst for knowledge, and a deep motivation to aid his fellow man. Unfortunately, today's stereotypical "premed" student seems altogether preoccupied with the former at the exclusion of the latter. While a good doctor must possess an innate intelligence and an ability to expand and update his knowledge, it is equally important that he or she be able to effectively interact and communicate with the co-workers and patients that surround him. I believe my experiences and accomplishments at Cornell show that I possess both the necessary desire and essential skills needed to succeed in the field of medicine.

In satisfying my thirst for knowledge, I have pursued a broad range of courses and employment that demonstrate my raw abilities. Science has always fascinated me, and I think my academic choices reflect those interests. In addition, I have acted as a research assistant for the past two summers under Dr. Stefan Cohen of the University of Buffalo Department of Medicine at Buffalo General Hospital, examining the tumoricidal effects of isolated liver cells. My work culminated with the acceptance of a paper, which I coauthored, entitled "Augmentation of Natural Cytotoxicity of Murine Nonparenchymal Liver Cells by Interferon or Interleukin 2" for publication this fall in *Sinusoidal Liver Cells* by Elsevier Biomedical Press.

To be an informed participant in contemporary society, though, requires more than just scientific intelligence and rote memorization. To fully appreciate that being we call man, one must have experience in the informed reflection upon the literature, philosophy, and art of our society, as well as an understanding of politics, history, and economics. The broad range of academic and extracurricular activities I have pursued in college demonstrates my desire to gain an extremely comprehensive exposure to such material, as well as the skills to solve problems and process information.

But knowledge in and of itself is insufficient. I perceive knowledge not as an end, but as a means to an end—helping people. A simple glance at the activities I have participated in at Cornell clearly illustrates how crucial others are to me, and I think there is one obvious conclusion—I like people! Whether it's teaching, helping, entertaining, talking, or just enjoying a good laugh, I am comfortable, confident, and effective interacting with other people. I am a member of the Delta Chi fraternity, where I have acted as Alumni Secretary, Corresponding Secretary, and a member of the Executive Board. I have been quite active as a College Ambassador, hosting potential students and giving tours to visitors at Cornell. I have also acted as a student advisor, advising students on various aspects of Cornell—whether it be scheduling problems or just roommate trouble. On campus I've held a number of jobs, and have also acted as a teaching assistant for an Oral Communications class. In addition, I am presently acting as a TA for both an Animal Physiology Laboratory and a Microcomputer Applications course. Each of these activities requires not only a considerable amount of responsibility, but a good deal of patience as well.

By far the most enjoyable (and time consuming) activites I am involved in have been singing with the Cornell Glee Club, and a small men's *a cappella* subset called the HANGOVERS—known both for our singing and our sense of humor. In more than three years of activity, we have toured California, the South Eastern U.S. and various portions of the Northeast, released an album, and performed for numerous gatherings of students, alumni, and friends, as well as the likes of Helmut Schmidt, Henry Kissinger, Gerald Ford, and Bob Hope.

Clearly, I have not allowed myself to become trapped in the static environment of the "preprofessional" student. I have managed to both expand my scope of knowledge and grow as an individual. Yet throughout this whole process I have also managed to focus my interests and intensify my desires. Without hesitation, I can honestly say that there can be no better choice for me than a career in medicine, for medicine combines the best of both worlds—working closely with people while continuing in a scientific field. I firmly believe I have the ability to succeed in such a career, and will find great satisfaction in patient care. Through a career in medicine I can help man at his most basic level, his physical presence, and still grow individually while contributing to society's wealth of knowledge.

While intent on pursuing an active practice, possibly in pediatrics, orthopedics, oncology, or geriatrics, I fully intend to incorporate both clinical and experimental research into my work. Farther down the road, I would like to become involved in public policy as it relates to health care and science. It seems fairly obvious that governmental legislation and policy has lagged far behind the advances being made in many scientific fields, and needs to be updated. While active medical practice is my primary goal, I feel that I could contribute significantly to both the scientific community and the general public by acting as as advocate for science among the politicians.

# Essay #28

Throughout the years I have spent in high school and college, my main career goal has been to become a physician. Although I have carefully examined many options, I feel that a career in medicine best suits my personal interests. Ever since I was a small child, I have had a special passion for biology. Understanding the various mechanisms and functions of the human body is my main biological interest. Through a thorough study and career in medicine, I believe that I will be able to satisfy my need to understand the various workings of the human system.

As a medical student and physician, I feel that I will be able to easily mix with the people who surround me. Being an only child (my 11-year old sister died when I was six years old), I was forced to interact with others in the community for social satisfaction. This enabled me to learn how to relate to a wide variety of people.

I have had a number of experiences with the medical profession, but my relationship with Dr. Henry Corn, a former family doctor now retired, sticks out most in my mind. Dr. Corn made patients feel at ease with his wit, humor, and compassion. His number one priority was the patient's health, and with this aspect, Dr. Corn was "strictly business." I feel that Dr. Corn was the epitome of the type of physician I will strive to be. It is important that doctors achieve a balance between subjectivity and objectivity. Through my experience observing Dr. Corn, I saw that he was a master at expressing proper concern for his patients, while not letting his concern get in the way of sound professional judgment.

Another person who has been a special influence to me is Herbert Hantz, my high-school English teacher. Mr. Hantz worked with me many times before and after school, teaching the importance of written expression as a complement to speech communication. He also instilled in me that there is honor and dignity in working hard to achieve goals. Even now, I call on Mr. Hantz from time to time to receive profitable advice and counsel.

During the summer before my first year of college, I had the opportunity to travel through Europe on a study tour with about thirty of my high-school classmates. In thirty-one days we traveled through the countries of Germany, Switzerland, Italy, France and England. This was the first time in my life that I met so many different people with varying cultural backgrounds. The trip helped me alleviate much of my ignorance about the world beyond America. Through socializing with the Europeans of differing countries, I learned the basic lesson that people are people wherever you go. Although there are many differences between the citizens of the world, we are all human beings experiencing joy, pain, anger and sorrow.

My commitment to medicine will be the largest factor affecting my success in the field. I have put a great deal of time and energy into seeking a medical career. Once this goal is obtained, my persistance will not subside. I feel that a physician is a public servant, one who must take the responsibility of giving that "extra effort" to insure that a patient gets the best medical care possible.

I firmly believe that I will make a viable contribution to the medical school to which I am accepted. I have the strength to carry on when the workload gets tough, and I also have the perseverence to weather setbacks that I will face. The school that accepts me will receive an excited student who will prove to the board of admissions that they did not make a mistake.

# Essay #29

It has been my ambition, for some time, to become involved in the medical profession. I chose medicine because I feel it is my duty in life to concern myself with the well being of others. This duty can best be fulfilled to my satisfaction by pursuing a career in medicine.

To fulfill my aspirations there are certain key qualities that I must acquire. I have begun to prepare for that responsibility by maintaining a strong academic background and involving myself in extracurricular activities and clinical experiences.

My undergraduate education has provided a strong background for my future studies in medical school. With a B.S. in Microbiology, I have acquired an indepth knowledge of the biological sciences. I have been able to improve my research and scientific skills by applying the knowledge to my Microbiology lab work with pathogenic organisms, such as *Neisseria gonnorhoae*.

The life of a good, dedicated physician involves more than knowing how the body functions. Equally important, is knowing how to deal with people on a personal basis. I have acquired some clinical experience in the area of interpersonal relationships. Two years ago I volunteered as a nurses aid at a local hospital. I worked primarily with elderly patients and became more sensitive to their special needs. This summer I am working as a volunteer in an Emergency Room. This experience has given me the opportunity to observe doctors and nurses in critical situations. I am also working with a doctor in his private practice. My duties involve filing charts, assisting patients, urine and stool analysis and developing X rays. I feel these experiences are invaluable to me in developing a sensitivity to patients and their needs.

My ethnic background has been a contributing factor in my prospective plan after medical school. I would like to work in a physician shortage area where a Puerto Rican background will be helpful in dealing with other hispanic minorities.

I want to succeed in my career goals. I will be a successful doctor if I am able to give the sick the compassion and quality medical care that they deserve.

# Essay #30

Simply stated, childhood accidents and subsequent visits to pediatricians, dentists, and hospitals established my interest in medicine. During these sessions, I was slowly exposed to many disciplines of practical medicine—radiology, anesthesiology, thoracic surgery, plastic surgery, emergency room medicine, and orthopedics. Although the visits themselves were not unusual for an active child, my enthusiasm may have been so; a broken bone presented another chance to see "how doctors worked".

As I grew, so did my enthusiasm for medicine. Fortunately, this fervor also matured. To my delight, I found that I didn't have to break an arm or step on a rusty nail to learn a little bit more about medicine. I turned rather to books, magazines, journals, and other sources of information. Very quickly, it was clear that medicine was not just doctors and hospitals but that it pervaded society in a very broad sense. With that realization, I began a scholastic, physical, and emotional approach to an eventual career in medicine.

During the second half of my freshman year at the University of Michigan, I applied for and was awarded a competitive pre-medical/medical scholarship through the United States Air Force. A part of this application required me to write a tentative plan of study for the following undergraduate years. This outline has served as the basis for my directed liberal-arts education. My studies have included subjects from molecular biology to astronomy and from comparative politics to the literature of Thomas Mann. This Summer, I have supplemented these studies with practical laboratory experience both fulltime in immunology under Dr. Latham Claflin and on a volunteer basis in Dr. Benedict Lucchesi's pharmacology laboratory.

Because I am most mentally fit when I am physically fit, my undergraduate years have also included a host of recreational and competitive sports. Regular tennis and squash matches as well as seasonal competition on the University of Michigan Rowing Team, therefore, have also contributed to my approach toward medicine.

Emotionally, there are both planned and unplanned events which prepare me for that side of medicine. Among those planned are challenging academic schedules as well as a year of study in Freiburg, West Germany. Occasionally, each of these examples was a source of stress and anxiety to be overcome. Planned psychological challenges, however, are often dwarfed by those not forecast. For many years, my father struggled to live with bipolar affective disorder and schizophrenia. As a family, we struggled with him. Last August, however, we had to involuntarily hospitalize him. He has since left our family. As the oldest of four children, I have been faced with both the loss of my father and a redefining of my role in the family. The events of this last year have caused me to question nearly everything I had taken for granted and have made me aware of unsuspected reservoirs of strength I had not known before.

I view my eventual career in medicine as one filled with both sacrifice and intangible reward. From broken bones and stepped-on rusty nails to directed collegiate years and unforseen tragedy, I have followed a pathway toward these sacrifices and gains. With all of the experiences which have prepared me for events to come, I anticipate four years of medical school with enthusiasm.

# Essay #31

The greatest motivational factor in my pursuit of a medical career was my work experience with the DuPont Company in the Cornell Engineering Co-Op Program. The seven months of research I performed at DuPont impressed upon me the similarities between my Chemical Engineering background and the increasingly technical nature of medicine. I was a member of a research group actively involved in improving certain types of polymers for industrial, as well as medical, applications. Polymers of this type find use in medicine due to their inert properties in the human body and other biological environments. As a research engineer, I also had the opportunity to learn about innovations within DuPont's Biomedical Products research laboratories. Here, I became aware of improvements in biotechnology and computers that will inevitably have a significant impact upon the quality of health care. Through this work experience in the engineering field, however, I also recognized that I wanted a career which places a greater emphasis on human relationships. A career in medicine will allow me to work with and help people in a more direct manner than I found possible in my engineering work.

As a student at Cornell University, I received a broad exposure to a variety of scientific disciplines which are the basis of many of today's rapidly advancing medical technologies. My interests in organic chemistry, biochemistry, and the engineering sciences were particularly important in forming my decision to enter a health-related career. I consider medicine to be a means for me to apply these or similar sciences in a most fulfilling and humane manner. In addition, I believe that the practical nature of my engineering education has afforded me a superior problem-solving ability that can be applied to medicine as well as other scientific fields.

After my formal education at Cornell, it was my intention to work two years in the engineering profession before entering medical school. During this time, I hoped to gain practical skills and management experience relevant to my future medical career. I worked for the Nestle Company following graduation as a manager-in-training in their food processing operations. At Nestle, I learned about the nutritional aspects of health and worked with people in my role as a supervisor.

After nine months with Nestle, I decided to accept another management position in mechanical design and manufacturing with the Ulster Tool and Die Corporation in Kingston, N.Y. My technical work at this firm, designing and developing specialized machinery, has given me the valuable knowledge of how people interact with mechanical devices. More importantly though, this opportunity to manage people in a professional environment has proven to be a most challenging and enjoyable task, confirming my decision to pursue a health career. The consistently high level of performance expected of me as a manager and engineer in this business has been an excellent preparation for my future responsibilities as a physician.

While being employed by Ulster Tool and Die, I have been performing volunteer work in the Radiology Department of the Benedictine Hospital in Kingston, N.Y. My work here, transporting and assisting patients for testing, has increased my familiarity with hospital procedures and proven to be a personally rewarding experience for me. From these practical pursuits in the hospital, working directly with patients and observing firsthand the realities of hospital life, I have had a candid introduction to health careers.

These varied experiences have given me the opportunity to more clearly define my professional goals. The time I have spent since my graduation from Cornell has been particularly important to me for personal growth and for making a more informed decision towards medicine. My strong background in the basic sciences, and the practical work experience I have in both the chemical industry and the hospital, have motivated me to pursue a health career.

To fulfill the medical school requirements, I completed the Biology requirement during the Summer of 1984 at Pace University. In order to accommodate the work schedule for the Cornell Engineering Co-Op Program, I completed the Fall 1982 semester's courses during the Summer of 1982. I worked for DuPont during the Fall of 1982 and the Summer of 1983. My participation in the Cornell Engineering Co-Op Program necessitated that I fulfill the organic chemistry requirement with the following sequence of courses: Organic Chemistry 253 (4 credit hours), Experimental Organic Chem. 251 (2 credit hours), and Industrial Organic Processes 421 (2 credit hours).

# Essay #32

I was born Dutch and spent the first nine years of my life in the Netherlands. At that time my father retired and took the family to France. We lived for fourteen years on the Swiss-French border outside of Geneva. The international atmosphere of Geneva was represented by the children at the International School of Geneva, where I was a student through high school. For example, one unique experience during high school was participating in the "Student United Nations". For three days students from several European schools acted as diplomats from the countries represented at the United Nations. The exposure and sharing of the varied culture, religions, traditions and languages has continued to help me to accept people for what they are and to be able to adjust more readily to diverse situations. By maintaining a certain level of academic achievement I was permitted to participate in sports. I enjoyed being a member of many teams especially, ski, basketball and track teams. I felt honored to be named sports woman of the year during my senior year. Although all sports brought me pleasure, skiing was my favorite. Therefore, I pursued it more intensely and eventually raced for the Dutch National ski team. At this level, skiing was demanding not only physically but also mentally. My memories of the pressure, losing as well as winning, but especially the comradery will always remain with me.

After high school I decided to continue my education at the University of Geneva. I had three particular interests, people, nature and sciences. Medicine was a serious consideration but due to the conservative attitude of my parents and Switzerland, the idea of a woman in medicine was not well supported. Without the obvious role models to look up to, I chose to study Biology. The University was rather academically oriented without emphasis on athletic or social activities. Nonetheless, I felt compelled to continue to compete in basketball, sailing and skiing. My last year of the University was spent involved in an independent research project in microbiology. The results of which were the basis of my thesis entitled "Analysis of the genetic polymorphism of the HLA-DRB genes coding for class II antigenes of the human histocompatibility complex". The research was fascinating and challenging but on the other hand I realized it was not as idealistic as I had imagined it to be. I liked the technology and knowledge involved in basic science but I found myself missing a more direct interaction with people.

That same year in the laboratory, I met the most wonderful man in the world who is now my husband. Mark was a Fulbright Scholar from the United States doing a year of research in Geneva. Fortunately, I completed my studies at the same time Mark finished his research. Therefore, I was able to go with Mark to the United States in August 1983 when he started at Cornell Medical School. It was my first time in the United States and the transition was made easier by Mark, his family and the fact that two of my best friends from high school happened to live in New York at the time. Since I was not yet a permanent resident it was initially difficult to find a job. After several waitressing jobs, a cardiologist hired me as his secretary. It was all new to me but I enjoyed the work, especially the patient contact. The atmosphere revived my old interest in medicine and I decided to continue my education. Again I considered medical school, but the surgical assistant program seemed like a perfect compromise. Being newly married a particular concern of mine was having the time for a family in the future. A shorter education with some responsibility and patient contact made the role of a surgical assistant look ideal. I loved learning about the applications of science in medicine, mastering some surgical techniques, and especially my interaction with the patients on the wards. Unfortunately, I soon realized that our short didactic course led us to become more technically oriented rather than problem solving members of the surgical team. I finally decided that I would never feel comfortable in this situation and that being an assistant would never satisfy me. Therefore, I quit the program to reevaluate my future plans.

This was not terribly difficult. By now I had had more exposure to the demands of medicine, what medicine represents, and had spent some time discussing the issues of women in medicine. Therefore, I now feel comfortable and excited about becoming a physician. So, with the support of Mark, I decided to pursue what deep inside I always wanted to do, apply for medical school.

# Essay #33

$W$hat kind of person would be insane enough to spend half of his life studying for a job which requires twelve hour work days, no vacations, and interminable patience — in other words total dedication? He must be a person who realizes the many responsibilities which such a prestigious, yet taxing vocation will require. Also, he must have observed the pride which a doctor feels when his patient is no longer dependent on others. I am such a person.

As a child, I was asthmatic. Though this never kept me from my daily romps through the mud on the way to school or from relishing every moment of gym class, I sometimes became ill at night. No matter what the hour, Dr. Orange would always come to the rescue, with a bag of medicine and a box of soothing words. Dr. Orange was my champion and I vowed to some day follow in his footsteps. This news was received enthusiastically by my parents who always encouraged my academic interests. Thus began my quest to become the first doctor in my family.

Although almost all of my hopes and dreams have changed since childhood, my longing to become a doctor has stood fast. My experience working at the Stanford VA Hospital has been a major force in solidifying this desire. I have been working in a psychopharmacology lab there for the past three years. I am very lucky to be a part of a lab in which I am treated as an equal with all other personnel, doctors, and researchers. I have become good friends with many of the doctors with whom I work. Whether it is during a three hundred tube assay or during a day of champagne tasting, I have seen the true life of a physician through the eyes of those who know: the politics involved, the hard work, and the great stress. Yet, I am a person who thrives on new and exciting challenges, and the thought of hard work does not have a negative connotation.

My own research has a taught me quite a lot as well. I am currently concluding my Human Biology honors project which I have been working on for the past year and am confident will be published this fall. It involves my testing the neurochemical and behavioral effects of a new drug, called Proglumide, to determine whether it can be used to treat Schizophrenia. Through this project I have learned to work on my own, solving problems which arose at the most inopportune times. I have become aware of the wealth of knowledge which one can acquire through hands on experience and by conversation with fellow research enthusiasts. I have experienced the humiliation and sense of helplessness one feels when an assay just will not work. Yet, I have also known the feeling of an incredible high when my first paper was published. I regard my research experience as one of the highlights of my undergraduate career. However, I like working with people, and I hope to experience the clinical side of medicine during my years in medical school; this will afford me the opportunity to decide exactly where I wish to put my energies during my years as a doctor.

What kind of person would go into medicine? A person who can endure the hardships in the hopes that one day he will hear the words, "Thanks Doc" from a patient who, a few hours earlier, could hardly breath, no less talk.

# Essay #34

$M$y activities at Cornell and in the Ithaca-Cayuga Heights communities are not preparations or exercises for a future way of life but are my way of life. Community service and working with people have always stimulated my daily experiences and have made my life more meaningful. The desire to make people's lives more tolerable and a penchant for scientific research are two qualities that can best be combined in a career in medicine. Thus, my motivations lie in the firm belief that I can make a considerable change in the human condition — for the better.

My medically related experience has been three-fold: volunteer hospital work, medical science research and ambulance service. First, at Bellevue, I worked in the Tumor Registry as the one responsible for interpreting patients' records and staging diagnosed cases of cancer. Although this was not a clinical experience, I learned a great deal of pathology, anatomy and medical terminology. I was also allowed to participate in Residents' discussions in the Ob.-Gyn. department next door where I became temporarily proficient at recognizing neoplastic cells and staging the endometrium from slides. This same summer, on alternate days, I volunteered as a research assistant, assisting a study on the pathology of cerebral brain ischemia in rats. This experience enabled me to sharpen my laboratory skills and understand the problems associated with medical research. Second, the next summer I conducted my own study investigating the lipid peroxide content of various foods under the supervision of M.L. Seligman, Ph.D. and H.B. Demopolous, M.D. (Klausner et al., J. Cornell Scientists, 1:1 and submitted J. Food Science). This study taught me about the value of preventative medicine, forced me to apply my knowledge of organic chemistry and familiarized me with the entire design of medical research from the conception of an idea to the publishing of the results. Third, I am a N.Y. State Certified Emergency Medical Technician and have served on a volunteer ambulance corps since 1980 and a rescue squad since 1983. These trauma experiences have been invaluable training for a career in medicine. I have learned how to stabilize patients through basic procedures and equally important how to inspire confidence in my coworkers.

My volunteer work with the Tompkins County 4-H includes

organizing weekly activities for a group of teenagers from the ages of 14-19. I use my Planned Parenthood training to educate them in contraception and offer frank sexual advice. I find this experience very rewarding and a welcome relief from the pressures at Cornell.

Being a member of Phi Kappa Sigma Fraternity has allowed me to exercise my great leadership and motivational abilities. The office of President gave me a chance to change the attitude and reputation of the Chapter from one of complacency and disorganization to activism and efficiency. Under my direction as Rush Chairman we were able to increase our new membership from an abysmal one in 1983-4 to eight in 1984-85 and I have been re-elected to this position for Fall 1985.

Perhaps my most interesting, at least my newest endeavor, was the creation and publication of the Journal of Cornell Scientists. I realized a lack of opportunities existed for undergradutes to publish research where their peers could read it and they could practice the format of scientific publication. The remedy was simple: to create such a journal on my own; however, the process was difficult and took a lot of ingenuity, Funds needed to be raised, a publisher found and submissions acquired. Within three months of the inception of the idea all three facets were readily realized and the first issue appeared in November, 1984.

The varied activities that I pursue indicate that I am a determined, motivated and conscientious individual, all essential qualities for a career in medicine. I perform well under pressure as any fellow firefighter will attest and get along remarkably well with youngsters, peers and elders. My future plans include incorporating my concern for human welfare, creativity and leadership abilities in becoming a surgeon, researcher and public policy official.

# Essay #35

During my years at Manhattan College, I have become determined in my desire to pursue a career in medicine. Condfident of my abilities and determination, I sincerely believe I possess the qualities to become a caring physician. Aside from academic achievement, I have demonstrated leadership qualities, intiative and an ability to empathize and to communicate with people.

At Manhattan College I chose to study electrical engineering because its stringent science curriculum would allow me to branch into other career fields. In my studies I have become aware of the many applications of electronic devices in medicine and I would like to apply my engineering education with a medical education to enable me to research and design or improve medical equipment. In order to learn more about medical application of electrical engineering, I have registered for a biomedical engineering course and am currently participating in a Manhattan College senior project in conjunction with the Orthontics and Prosthetics Department of New York University Medical Center designing electric circuitry to improve the N.Y.U. Hosmer Prosthetic Elbow.

As a member of Eta Kappa Nu, National Honor Society of Electrical Engineers, I served as a tutor for other electrical engineering students and participated in the design, construction and presentation of an electrical stimulator to reduce muscle pain for Manhattan College Open House ceremonies. I was selected to New York Zi Chapter of Tau Beta Pi, National Engineering Honor Society, and am currently serving on the chapter Executive Board and selection committee and represent the chapter at district events.

At Manhattan College I served as a group leader in the Freshman Orientation Program. Later, I was selected to serve in their Peer Counselor Program in which upper classmen offer peer assistance and direction to freshman through the semester, beginning with general orientation and including weekly group meetings and work-shops on study habits and test anxiety. Since freshman year, I have been an active member of Alpha Phi Delta National Fraternity, serving as a member of the Judiciary Committee, Intramural Chairman, Pledgemaster and chapter organization. I have helped organize and have participated in many charity fund raising events for organizations such as the American Heart Association, Special Olympics and the American Cancer Society and have also participated in a program with the Methodist Church Home for the Aged, spending time with the elderly people at the home. The ability to communicate and work with others has been an essential element of much of my activities at Manhattan College.

For the past seven years I have worked at Carvel Ice Cream Store No. 699 on Staten Island and have served as a weekend and night manager for the past four years. The money I have earned together with my scholarship and student loan has helped pay for my college expenses. In the summer following my sophomore year, I volunteered in the emergency room of Bayley Seton Hospital on Staten Island. This enabled me to observe medical professionals at work and to understand the dedication and teamwork necessary for successful patient care.

I recognize that many factors must be considered in choosing medical students. I am confident that my background in academics, extracurricular activities, community involvement and personal commitment fulfill the qualifications you seek in applicants.

# Essay #36

I have always been interested in science and have practiced studio art and have wrestled for ten years. But it is difficult to expain my interest in three such widely differing pursuits as part of an underlying state of mind. After some thought, I was surprised to realize that there is indeed a similar motivation for all three activities.

This motivation relates to a deep interest I have always had in mythology and science fiction. The stories that most appeal to me are of individuals alienated from, or cast into, an alien society, struggling to assert their independence and individuality. By suspending my disbelief, I can partake in the struggle of the fictional characters and feel their victories and defeats. Art, wrestling and science are all, in a sense, isolating activities, and each requires a great deal of discipline and training. One cannot paint a picture the first time one steps into a studio; nor can one wrestle well the first time on a mat. Research requires the patience to gather the proper data, and also creativity to interpret the data correctly. These three interests have served as my way of becoming in reality the adventurers I have read about.

Let me elaborate. Several months ago, I was busy writing my thesis. I have already spent the better part of a year gathering data and running assays in a laboratory, and all that was left was the interpretation of the data. I found that instead of dreading the long hours of writing and rewriting, I looked forward to it. I felt that I was fitting in the final pieces of a large jigsaw puzzle or coming to the end of an intricate detective story, and it was exciting to watch the overall picture slowly emerge. The feeling, surprisingly, was akin to a feeling I often get whenever I draw an excellent picture or wrestle a perfect match. In all these instances, I achieve a certain rhythm and feeling of inspiration that enables me to work with a minimum of energy. It is said that long distance runners experience a feeling called "runners' high," that makes them addicted to their running. The high I experience when I wrestle and win a match, draw an excellent picture or piece together bits of research is just as addictive. When I read science fiction, I identify with the protagonist because I feel that the control and effort vital to their successes are similar to qualities in myself that enable me to spend ten hours straight working on a picture, or spend weeks preparing for a wrestling match.

I have always wanted to be a doctor because I have sensed that much of a doctor's work will satisfy me in the way that my other interests satisfy me. I am careful, however, not to confuse my love of adventure and fantasy with my reasons for wanting to be a physician. For a long time I had conceived of myself as going through the medical training process so that I could become a "doctor/hero." Wielding a shining scalpel, I would cure all of my patients' problems with stunning success. What I now realize is that for most of my future patients, there will be no one sure method of treatment, and many of them may not respond to treatment at all.

Thus, it is my feeling that a doctor should be more than a dispenser of health care; he should also take an active role in the health community. It seems to me that the rising cost of health care and increasingly bewildering technology have created a breach in the rapport between doctors and the public. Many patients feel that they have little control or understanding of their treatment. As a doctor, I may not be able to cure or even help all of my patients, but, if I can help to bridge the gap between my and my patients' knowledge, then I will be as satisfied as I ever was reading myths and fiction. When I am a physician, I feel that the discipline and control I have learned from my other interests will serve me well, but more importantly I feel that the enthusiasm and joy that I derive from these interests will also be an internal part of my life as a doctor. Hopefully, my future patients will sense my enthusiasm and be encouraged by it.

# Essay #37

Although I have learned a great deal through formal course work, this has provided only a part of my education. During the past year, I have had the opportunity to work in an operating room (Summer '84) and an emergency room (Winter '84- Spring '85) of hospitals at home and at college. Although quite different, both were valuable learning experiences. In the operating room, I was able to observe how the hospital staff worked together in performing the mechanics of an operation. The emergency room, on the other hand, allowed me to see the impact that illness had on the patient and those close to him. These experiences have taught me that in addition to mastering the technical skills, success is dependent on the personal qualities of the physician. These qualities include compassion, emotional strength, and the ability to instill confidence in people.

I have developed some of these personal qualities in my work as a camp counselor for underprivileged children (Summer '83) and as a Big Brother (1983-84) to a young boy living near my college. These experiences have also allowed me to know the feeling of having people depend on me, which is an important aspect of being a physician.

This summer I am working in a laboratory at The Sloan-Kettering Cancer Institute. I have always had a strong interest in research. I believe that investigative work helps build an inquiring, independent, and analytical approach to learning while developing the ability to evaluate and solve problems with ingenuity. The rapid therapeutic advances of today make this an asset, not only in academic careers such as medical research and teaching, but in clinical practice as well.

My parents are physicians so I have always been exposed to the field of medicine, a field which has interested me for much of my life. The past few years have provided opportunities for me to test this interest and strengthen my decision to pursue a career in medicine. It is a career which I am confident will provide numerous challenges and a lifetime of learning.

# Essay #38

As a person who is highly interested in the sciences and in people, a career in medicine has always appealed to me. The ability to heal the sick is a gift I hope to attain and put to use. As time passes, I am more eager to become a surgeon and to practice medicine in or near a large city.

My first medical related experience occurred in the summer after my sophomore year of high school. I participated in the American Foundation for Negro Affairs Program (AFNA). This program supported the idea that more minorities were needed in the medical profession and financed tours of medical schools, showed filmstrips of surgical procedures, and presented lectures by medical doctors. AFNA increased my interest in medicine tremendously and was a major influence in my decision to become a doctor.

During my junior year, I became a volunteer worker at Lafon Nursing Home in New Orleans where I worked closely with the nurses and residents. This not only required me to learn several duties of nursing, but also taught me to become patient, understanding, and perservering in dealing with others.

The following summer I attended the Stress on Analytical Reasoning Program (SOAR) at Xavier University. Its purpose is to prepare incoming students for science and math courses. This program was the final determining factor in my becoming a Chemistry major at Xavier University.

In the sumer of 1982, prior to entering Xavier, I became a volunteer worker at Louisiana State Medical School in New Orleans. As a result, I participated in research studies pertaining to cancer as an inherited disease. In addition, I actively participated in the growth of amniotic fluid cell cultures which helped me to learn the importance of cleanliness and sterile equipment.

At Xavier, I am a member of various social organizations and academic honor socities. At the end of my sophomore year, a decision was made to become less involved in extracurricular activities and to focus my energies on my courses. As a result, I completed the junior year, my hardest year as a Chemistry major, even more motivated than before. The science courses that I have taken left me fascinated with the structure and systems of the human body. I wish to continue my quest for knowledge in medical school, to further my understanding of how the body functions.

While attending Xavier, I also held a job as a student lab assistant in the hematology department of Charity Hospital in New Orleans. For two years I worked approximately twenty-five hours a week and became very familiar with the operations of this department. I tested blood for sickle cell anemia and learned how to do retic counts, but became most experienced in urinalysis. In addition, I was able to see how doctors are viewed by other hospital personnel.

Intrinsically, I am highly motivated. Extrinsically, I have a loving supportive family and the confidence of the highly competent faculty of Xavier. Together, the above supply me with the confidence, courage and knowledge needed not only to attend medical school, but also to succeed. Having spent the last several years of life preparing to learn how to help the sick and the needy, I feel that my talents can best be exercised by becoming a doctor and working to heal others. This is my goal in life.

# Essay #39

As a child I believed that the answer to the polite old question of what would I like to do when I grow-up was a simple one. One just chose what one did best, most naturally and loved the most. It seemed so easy to answer; I would grow-up and help people. Although my basic approach had a lot of truth to it, my naivete of the complexities of decision-making is apparent. Knowledgeable decisions require more than just good instinct.

All the truly important resolutions in our lives require time and care. Benjamin Franklin used to sit and write out the pros and cons of each problem before arriving at a decision. He gave each reason a rating which he then tallied for an answer carrying the highest score. This process gave him the opportunity to identify the really weighty issues and allowed him to take the wisest course.

As a thoughtful individual I can appreciate Franklin's approach as I have come to live the pros and cons which have led me to my recent career-decision. My desire to study medicine was born out of my attempts to understand and help people and my pursuit of the discipline of psychology.

I have studied many perspectives in psychology and the more I learned the more I realized that the field had too narrow a focus on people. It really addressed only half the issue of human development by virtually ignoring the biological aspects of human behavior. Understanding the whole individual means learning about both the psychological and biological facets since neither is complete without the other. Having recognized this vital link between the two fields, I have actively dedicated myself to pursuing a career that encompasses both disciplines.

I have never let go of my interest in people. To really excel and truly appreciate my career choice, I have held on to my youthful ideal of identifying with that special quality of helping people which comes so naturally to me. While some would be reluctant to change course, I have welcomed the challenge and allowed my experience in psychology to help me clearly define my goals. I, unfortunately, took chemistry at a time when it had little relevance in my life; psychology had consumed my interest. I missed most of the classes and should have dropped the course; a mistake that I hope is one of very few.

By taking the time to explore and better organize my skills, I have also been able to make a knowledgeable and intellectually sound decision.

# Essay #40

$S$ome of my foremost objectives in the past three years have been to obtain a "well rounded" education, determine the benefits of a medical career, and to prepare myself adequately for such a career. By choosing a social science (economics) as a major and by working in research labs at the University of Minnesota (Minneapolis) Medical School during the past three summers, I believe I have attained all three goals. My transcript and recommendations attest my progress in the first goal. In the remaining essay, I will comment on my progress in the latter two.

Having witnessed a limited sample of the routines of physicians at the University of Minnesota hospital during the past three summers, I think one of the greatest satisfactions of practicing medicine would be correctly diagnosing a patient, prescribing an effective treatment, and observing the patient's recovery. Moreover, a physician would be able to reap these benefits daily.

In the long run though, I would like to be a physician who researches medicine on a "basic science" level and, at the same time, translates advances in scientific theory into clinical practice. I have spent the past two summers working on projects which, at first, do not appear applicable to current medical problems, but may eventually help lead to new clinical treatments. For example, last summer I researched the effects of human fibrinogen on the phagocytosis of *Escherichia coli* by human polymorphonuclear neutrophils (PMNs). My study revealed that an indirect relationship exists between fibrinogen concentration and phagocytic killing by neutrophils. This conclusion might appear interesting but clinically of little value; it may, however, help elucidate the mechanism by which fibrin clots inhibit phagocytosis of *E. coli* by neutrophils. Hence, a treatment could be developed which might prevent the formation of peritoneal abscesses and intraabdominal sepsis. An accomplishment like this would be, I believe, of great and lasting satisfaction.

Presently, I am working on a project studying the effects of hyperoxia on cutaneous wounds. The literature reveals that when an inoculum of *E. coli* is injected intradermally with a mass inoculation gun into a guinea pig, the resultant lesion will be smaller if the animal is contained in a hyperoxic environment. The literature, so far, makes no reference to a mechanism. To

identify this mechanism is the object of my current investigation.
The research hypothesis loosely reads, "increased partial pressures of oxygen in the ambient air lead to a more effective exidative burst on the part of the neutrophils; thus, bacteria are cleared from the wound more quickly, and the wound can heal faster." The practical applications of this project are more readily apparent than in my previous research. People with cutaneous wounds could be treated more effectively with the administration of oxygen. Again, an advancement in the understanding of a basic science problem, such as wound healing, would have been translated into clinical practice. Satisfactions such as this are one of my main reasons for choosing medicine.

# Essay #41

**P**raeludium. In the beginning there was dissonnance. The lifeless world was still and silent. Then God breathed life unto man, giving realm of his own. And then one night, man was given the power to create, to discover and to question. And as he created fire to heal him from the cold he discovered the sound of the flickers generated by his fire-maker. Like Apollo's Lyre when forged by Hermes, man's instrument was imbued with the magic of life. The magic to heal him from the cold he called medicine. The magic to create new sounds which brought him internal warmth he called music . . . Undoubtedly, music and medicine were born on the same day. From Apollo, who is god of both, to Johannes Brahms' best friend and trusted critic, the famous surgeon Theodore Billroth, music and medicine have courted each other incessantly. I am in love with both.

**Allegro ma non troppo.** My love for music is more than the desire to compose, interpret and listen; like my love for medicine is more than the desire to conduct research, practice and study. Rather, I wish to understand these two worlds, to internalize their principles so they become second nature to me, for love alone is not enough. I have not always felt this way: I decided to pursue medicine only after my second year in college. And music was not very exciting to me when I was sixteen. Unrelated yet similar incidents propelled me into these realms. I don't really know how it happened, but one day while playing the piano, I decided to improvise. As I played new combinations of notes, I felt free, uninhibited. Needless to say my improvisations soon became compositions. Discovering that I could be original, treading on my own musical road was one of the greatest gifts of life, because it radically modified my approach to music. In medicine it happened differently. During my first 2 years in college I wished to become a biochemical researcher, but a key factor unknown to me was missing. During spring break I volunteered to do social work in a small Mexican village. With some romanticism I observed the village physician work with his rudimentary instrumentation healing, teaching and mainly learning in this isolated Shangri-La. Like with music, I learned that this physician could heal in his own creative way and be rich in spite of this town's emptiness. Doing this required creativity and openness. However I made many mistakes after that because I asked what if . . . I only compose? What if I study only medicine?

**Andante.** Soon after beginning to compose, my piano skills were weakened and I found myself lacking discipline. Eventually, my composition ceased because there was no knowledge on which to base my ideas. Similarly, I began to doubt my studies at Stanford. It seemed so much easier to return to Mexico where one begins medical school after high school . . . In music and medicine there exists a fine artistic domain which permits individual expression, care and much subjectivity. Yet this freedom can subsist because there is a rigid framework supporting and fueling it. To the composer this freedom is the realm of emotions. In the medical world this artistic domain is expressed in the individuality of each person. Often, even in what appears to be straight procedural medicine, one finds room for subjectivity. I once translated for a urologist with a Spanish—speaking patient. She had been preliminarily diagnosed with kidney stones and came to see a specialist. The urologist began with an interview rather than a physical. As he progressed he soon discovered that the patient's husband was abusing her both sexually and physically. No kidney stones were found and she was subsequently treated by a therapist. I was inspired by this physician's ability to seek alternate explanations, literally outside his area of expertise. But he was able to carry this freedom because his understanding of medicine is so complete, and so profound. So I decided to study harmony and develop a deeper understanding of music. It then became evident to me that Stanford was the right choice. Perhaps the common bond between music and medicine is their dual nature. There seems to be no clear border between the artistic and the scientific aspects of either. The famous composer Shoenberg once said that everything of supreme value in art must show "heart" as well as "brain". Perhaps this is the most important lesson I have learned: to use my subjective freedom better by strengthening its fundamental base. When I began my research on eating disorders I was given much freedom, being able to design studies entirely by myself. The only given was the issue to address. At that point I began to cherish the vast resources of the medical library, in strengthening my knowledge. In music, when I began to play the flute, I decided to focus on technique rather than feeling. And I have learned more about both in the last year, than ever before. With the flute I have also discovered the joys of multi-instrumental music, chamber music. The ideal medical team should be like a chamber ensemble, each contributing to the whole, yet not drowning the others or becoming impersonal. I would like to practice thus.

   **Adagio.** Important as music is to me, I have not considered music vocationally. Mainly for one reason: even though I love to perform, and write music for others, music plays a selfish role in my life. It challenges my senses and intelligence, and often it heals me, yet I cannot offer my knowledge to others. Medicine offers me many of the same challenges and satisfactions that music does, yet throughout I know that I can act for others as well. This is vital to me. In the past few weeks I have suffered because of the earthquake in my Mexico City. That day, especially, there was no room for music, only for medicine and I grieved for my lack of knowledge.

   **Allegro con spirite.** Whenever I study a musical piece I study the biography of the composer. I believe that music always reflects the personality of the composer. Sometimes it reflects temporal feelings; others it reflects the composer's constant views on life. I choose to believe this because my music is entirely human. I write music for people, and sometimes write about people; but I always write as a human. In the same way I choose to believe that medicine is primarily human. It is very easy to lose track of this, especially while doing research, when one thinks in terms of enzymes and tRNA. I like to see both music and medicine in "Gestalt" terms. As I face my instrument, myriads of combinations flash across my mind and I visualize the harmonic implications of many, yet I cannot explain how I piece my notes together. Something deeper which I know not is ever present in my style. In medical terms, I've observed this in Anorexia Nervosa. This disorder is treated by some with pure psychology, others treat it as a physiological sickness. Yet there's much more to it. On one level there exists social pressure, family problems etc.; but deeper there must be a physiological mechanism which operates concurrently with the rest. One world influences the other resulting in a deadlocked circle. Subtle feelings which permeate my harmony, of the subtle biochemical processes that transcend the purely psychological; always knowing that this is life I am dealing with. Music and medicine have no lives of their own. Man gives them life so that they might celebrate his life. My flute lies before me, inorganic, not even latent. And yet I breathe life unto it and it speaks, sings, soothes. So lies my profession before me, and I can hardly wait to breathe life unto it so that it may in turn speak, sing, soothe and heal, breathing new life unto others.

# Essay #42

Senior year at The Spence School, I discovered how inter-related the sciences could be. Understanding the basis of computer function and its similarities to the electrochemical nature of the nervous system, I realized how interesting the study of nature would be, especially with regards to the human system.

The summer following graduation I worked in the lab of Dr. P. R. Smith studying protein structure through electron microscopy. I was amazed how such research was based on basic principles within my grasp. I also began to realize how research on a day-to-day basis evolves rather than explodes, progressing by a series of smaller steps and variations on known procedures. The entire process seemed more like creative "playing" than work, despite the vast amount of knowledge behind each new variation. For two summers I worked in this lab developing a procedure to record electron micrographs of rotated crystals making possible 3-D reconstruction of the protein.

The following two summers I worked for Dr. Robert D. Allen at the Marine Biological Laboratory in Woods Hole. Dr. Allen was a role model in both professional and personal aspects. In the lab Dr. Allen had perfected the art of "playing" with a specimen and allowed me free rein to do the same. It was here I learned the value of "playing" with a specimen (in educated ways) in order to obtain the desired result. Our attempts to disturb the microtubules in extruded axoplasm resulted in our paper on "gliding microtubules" (1985). Outside the lab Dr. Allen expressed his creativity in his cello performances. I began to see how deciphering a biological system was comparable to figuring out a "harmony". I also enjoy both listening to and performing music and hope to strike a rewarding balance between personal and professional creativity as Dr. Allen did.

The two summers I spent at MBL had a profound effect on my approach to my studies and instilled in me a desire to learn as much as possible. Surrounded by distinguished scientists and taking advantage of daily lectures, I came to realize that learning is a privilege. My ability to grasp difficult concepts improved with my increased exposure to new fields.

During these summers of research, however, I realized how important human interactions are to me. In high school I spent two years helping my grandmother through the difficulties associated with age. After she died, I enjoyed helping the elderly at holiday dinners organized by our church. In losing my closest grandparent, I gained several hundred more. In grade school my father sustained multiple heart attacks and during my sophomore year he suffered a stroke. The following year was made more difficult when both my aunt and Dr. Allen developed cancer. During this period I began to see how illness and medicine related to the sciences I had been studying, and I realized this was the field I was most interested in pursuing.

I returned to Amherst determined to put my knowledge into my senior research project. In order to devote myself totally to this goal, I decided to wait a year before applying to medical school. My experience with and love of photography played a major role in our success as my aesthetic sense and desire to get good photographs of beautiful cells constantly led us to better pictures and an abundance of cytological information we had not expected.

While I have participated in research over the last four years, I have seen its applications help my own family. I would therefore gain satisfaction from involvement in both the research aspect of medicine and its practical applications in patient care.

# Essay #43

My goal for wanting to attend medical school is not to become just another M.D. but instead to become a warm and caring physician who is willing and able to humbly serve the people and their community to bring about improvements for the present human condition. In order to accomplish such task one must have the necessary dedication, knowledge and love for others.

Dedication to a worthy goal is important because this is what enables one to accomplish things beyond the ordinary limit. In whatever one does, without dedication, he can only reach mediocrity. This summer, through the help of the U.C.C. (United Church of Christ), I had the opportunity to dedicate my vacation to working as a volunteer at a missionary hospital in a small town called Humacao in Puerto Rico. While working there I've gained practical experience in different departments of the hospital. The most learning experience was working as a physician's assistant at their Home Care Program. In this program, health care professionals commute for hours to reach isolated households in the countryside to give treatment to those poor patients who can not get to the hospital themselves. From working with these dedicated physicians I realized that a strong sense of dedication is the driving force that pushes one to achieve deeds that are beyond the limit of an ordinary doctor. That is why I want to become a humble, compassionate doctor who is sincerely dedicated to improving the human condition.

However, with dedication alone I can not accomplish this task; I need the necessary skills and knowledge which will enable me to take actions toward my goal. During my years at Cornell, I've concentrated on getting a well-rounded liberal education rather than a science-oriented premedical education. I've tried to study as many courses in humanities and social sciences as I could, and I'm also majoring in Spanish literature because I believe one must first be a well-rounded human being who can think before he can become a competent worker in any field of profession. Knowledge is not knowing a lot of scientific facts and data, but instead it's the ability to think creatively and analytically, the power of observation and problem solving, and the infinite curiosity to discover the unknown. This year I'll be doing undergraduate research on lipid biochemistry because I believe that exploring into what is unknown is equally impor-

tant as mastering what is already known. I want to become a
kind of a doctor who will expand the horizon of the current
medical knowledge because the never-ending desire to understand the inexplicable is the key to the progress of the world.

Dedication and knowledge are indispensable elements in the
making of a warm and caring physician; however, they are not
sufficient. In order to become a "complete" doctor who is competent, compassionate and understanding, one must be able to
love the mankind. In the future I want to become a loving doctor who has a warm, family-like relationship with each and
every one of his patients, the kind of a doctor who can readily
communicate and understand his patients on one-to-one basis
because such doctor-patient communication is invaluable in
treating a patient. During my undergraduate years I've been
involved in a wide range of extracurricular and community activities from which I've learned a lot about human relations.
I've also worked overseas where I've been exposed to different
people and culture. From these experiences I've gained the patience, understanding and a caring heart, all of which are
necessary in communcating and dealing with all kinds of difficult people and situation, and I believe this qualification will
help me greatly in becoming a compassionate and understanding
doctor who can readily meet the needs of the people.

# Essay #44

My desire to become a physician originated during my childhood, a time when my father, who is himself a physician, served as my primary mentor and role model. As I matured, the initially blind longings he instilled in me were transformed into apprised aspirations and viable expectations. I have come to esteem medicine as a dynamic field promising a career filled with challenge and change. In addition, it offers the opportunity to have a positive impact on society while insuring a measure of respect and financial security. Equally appealing to me are medicine's clinical aspects, for I greatly value the chance to interact with a varying mix of people in diverse situations.

That these elements are indeed important career expectations for me has been self-substantiated by numerous personal experiences. Growing up in a family of seven, I have known all my life the pleasures of cooperation and interhuman relationships. In addition, my many years of participation in team sports have increased my proclivity for group interaction, as have my more recent experiences living with twenty other individuals in my fraternity house. This need for close contact and association with people has always been a prominent facet of my personality, and it is one I hope will find continued expression through clinical medicine.

I have also always felt the need to be challenged, and this has afforded me some very gratifying experiences. Entering college I had no prior exposure to secure myself a spot in the Crew program. This led to two very enjoyable seasons of rowing, and allowed me to develop some close friendships in addition to the techniques and skills of a new sport. Sportscasting was also foreign to me prior to college, but over the past three years I have managed to work my way up to the senior position among hockey commentators at the college radio station. This pursuit has not only proved to be exciting, but also quite beneficial as it has improved my extemporaneous oratory skills.

I have also tried to challenge myself academically at college, and this pledge bolstered my resolution to undertake study of the Chinese language. While these have perhaps been my most difficult courses, they have also been my most enjoyable. From them I have developed a fascination with the Chinese culture which not only has led me to major in this area, but, beginning this summer, I will undertake an intensive three month course of study in the People's Republic of China, followed by an additional three months of study in Taiwan. It is my hope that these next six months will not only afford me fluency in the Chinese language, but an intimate look at an alien culture and the opportunity to augment my intellectual and emotional growth, as well.

Though limited by space, it is my hope that these few preceeding examples demonstrate my commitment to the characteristics of a career in medicine. Furthermore, I have strengthened this commitment through extensive service as a hospital volunteer. Since high school I have worked at different hospitals in patient transport, intensive care, and pediatrics. My current volunteer work playing with hospitalized children typifies the whole range of these experiences. The immediate emotional gratification I receive from my work, though tempered by an often brutal reality, has made my attraction towards medicine even more genuine and concrete.

As I conclude, a Confucian aphorism comes to mind: "The wise embrace all knowledge, but they are most earnest about what is of the greatest importance." Throughout college I have been diligent in embracing many different streams of knowledge. However, graduation necessitates an estimation of these varied intellectual pursuits, and, for me, there is little question that, among them, my ambition to study medicine ranks supreme.

# Essay #45

"**I**f you don get paid, why the Hell do you work here?"
While working at the Pine Street Inn, Boston's largest
shelter for the homeless, this question came up often. Before
giving an honest answer, one is forced to do a lot of
soul searching. I could have, after all, chosen a more pleasant
placement than the Inn, where for ten hours a week I comforted and assisted hundreds of alcoholic and often deeply
disturbed individuals. These derelicts shared a misery too
profound for words.

In such an atmosphere of despair and frustration, one must
still try to find some achievement for your own piece of mind,
while dealing with a social system that has completely failed
these individuals. The Inn teaches you to strive for improvement no matter how small, and even though so much is needed. In trying your best at whatever you do, it is important to
understand your own limitations, both personal and within the
system. Several times I've spent hours talking to a "guest",
and have left the Inn beaming with a sense of accomplishment
only to be discouraged when a week later my new friend is on
the floor, quiet in unconsciousness except for an occasional
cough from lungs that only God could have designed to last
through such punishment. Compassion is born in places like
this, and can possess you totally if not kept in perspective.

A physician's practice in many ways parallels this experience.
His limitations are the scientific laws governing our bodies.
When fighting for another's life becomes your vocation, losing
to death becomes a hard pill to swallow. Our knowledge of
medicine is ever growing, yet the nemesis of death will always
be the final victor.

Why ride an emotional rollercoaster and volunteer at the
Pine Street Inn, or dedicate yourself to becoming a physician?
Because in helping people, you gain an understanding and
compassion that sensitizes you to a wide range of human
conditions, and makes you want to do your share in trying to
better them.

# Essay #46

I was born in Hungary and received a well-rounded education complete with 10 years of extra-curricular piano, singing, ballet and language lessons. From an early age I was fascinated by the scientific and technological advances of the West to the extent that I decided to emigrate and, at the age of 12, began to study English in preparation for this move. I received a Ph.D. in Psychobiology from Eotvos Lorand University in Budapest in 1977 and left for the U.S.A. the same year.

I received a post-doctoral fellowship at the Neurology Department of the University of Pennsylvania Medical School. Here I learned about various brain imaging techniques such as Positron Emmission Tomography (PET), Nuclear Magnetic Resonance and regional Cerebral Blood Flow and developed a strong interest in functional neuroanatomy. I devised a PET study which demonstrated an asymmetry of glucose metabolism in the human posterior parietal lobes during the performance of directed attentional tasks. Furthermore, I demonstrated an asymmetry of cortical control of heart rate in humans under conditions of unilateral barbituration of the hemispheres. Neither of the above had been previously reported in the literature. I was also involved in projects studying the impact of cognitive tasks on cerebral glucose metabolism, glucose metabolism changes in epilepsy and in schizophrenia.

In 1982 I was invited to present my findings at Behavioral Neurology Grand Rounds at Beth Israel Hospital of Harvard Medical School and was offered a 2 year NIH institutional National Research Service Award. At Harvard I worked on a study describing the distribution of acetylocholinesteraze in the primate cortex and a study describing the cortico-cortical connectivity of the temporal poles of primates. I also had the opportunity to attend Neurology Grand Rounds and Behavioural Neurology Grand Rounds on a weekly basis for 2 years. This experience was my first exposure to brain lesioned patients and it made me realize that clinical observation is perhaps the richest source of information in the study of neuroanatomical correlates of human behaviour. I found the clinical experience intellectually fascinating as well as emotionally stimulating and it triggered a strong desire in me to become a physician.

Two years ago I enrolled in the post-baccalaureate pre-medical program of Hunter College. Last year I had the singular honour of being placed at the top of the list of accepted candidates at both the Cornell and Mount Sinai Medical School linkage programs. I have chosen the Cornell program due to its newly established PET facility as well as its exceptional reputation in the neurosciences.

# Essay #47

Before coming to Brandeis, my decision to pursue a medical career was based solely on my interest in the sciences. However, my experiences over the past three years have been very self revealing, and not only has my reasoning for pursuing a medical career been modified, but also the type of career which I plan to pursue.

My extracurricular and work experience at Brandeis have helped me to realize both my desire to interact and work with others and my skill and ability to do so. As captain of both intramural football and basketball teams, I voluntarily placed upon myself an added responsibility. While this responsibility was at times a slight burden, I found that being captain made the overall experience more challenging and exciting. Working at Brandeis for the past two years as a chemistry group tutor has also enabled me to interact with and instruct others. Occasionally this became a humbling experience after struggling with a problem or concept with which I was not familiar. However, the gratitude expressed by the students, and my own ability to grapple with the problems, almost always made it rewarding and worthwhile.

In addition to my work at Brandeis, I spent the past two summers working at The Rockefeller University in Manhattan in a biochemistry lab. Last summer I was given an independent research project involving the determination of the metabolism of a certain super androgen. I found it to be a fascinating educational experience, and I learned firsthand the manner in which biomedical research is done and the many frustrations and obstacles which inherently go along with it. My summer work has been very inspirational. This summer I will begin my senior honors research in biochemistry for which I was awarded the Doris Brewer Cohen Award. I now plan on doing research as part of my career. However, working in the lab has also made me realize that I do not want to do research exclusively. At times I felt somewhat isolated, and I believe that I would be better suited in a career which would integrate research and application of my scientific knowledge to real life situations.

My decision to pursue a medical career now has a much more solid foundation upon which to build. I believe that my desires and talents will be best fulfilled and utilized in a medical career which involves both research and clinical work.

# Essay #48

Several incidents, over the past five years, have been major influences on my decision to become a physician.

I recall performing an emergency test on a boy suspected of having appendicitis. The next morning I encountered his mother, and was struck by the look of concern on her face. This made me realize the importance of the contribution I had made to the attempt to save the boy's life.

Even though I found working as a technician gratifying, an event occured that made me want to participate more meaningfully in the care of patients. While working in a medically underserved area, I performed a test for bleeding and clotting time on a man with a snake-bite. The patient died because of the unavailability of a doctor. Watching the dead man I felt a strong sense of inadequacy because, even though I had known the test results were abnormal, I could do nothing to help the patient. I decided to pursue a career that would enable me to make a greater contribution to the care of patients.

One experience as a resesarch aide gave me some appreciation of how doctors might feel when faced with a frustrating situation, and how they might deal with such a situation. After working on a synthesis of a labelled amino acid for several weeks, I isolated a product that was totally unexpected. I felt frustrated and defeated. After careful examination I discovered that the reaction mechanism was different from the one proposed. I had actually discovered the true reaction mechanism. This experience taught me that regardless of your hard work and dedication, there will always be instance of failure, and the best way to deal with these failures is to use them as learning experiences.

Three aspects of my character that I consider important are my self-discipline, my ability to relate to others, and my honesty. Honesty to myself is of special importance because it enables me to identify my strengths and weaknesses, and to be aware of my limitations.

I am confident that I will be able to function well as a physician because of my character, and the experience I have acquired. I have been exposed to various aspects of health care, and I am comfortable working in a hospital environment. Having worked on call I have learned to deal with the stress of making crucial decisions quickly and working long hours with little or no sleep. Thus, I can begin to appreciate the demands a career in medicine will make on me. However, I know it is what I want, and I am willing to work hard to succeed.

# Essay #49

I worked in the observatory this summer as a computer programmer. Working in programming was a valuable learning experience but even more valuable was observing the interaction between people in the maintenance staff, the technical staff, and the scientific staff. It was often interesting to see how important was all their work to keep the observatory running smoothly. I will relate what I observed during one of my days of work.

This day was very important for one of the scientists. After about five to six years of planning an experiment, the day for performing the experiment had arrived. The experiment was done in conjunction with the Space Shuttle. At about midnight the Shuttle would boost its engines right above the radio-telescope; gasses from the engines would disturb the ionosphere making a hole in it. This disturbance would be observed from the telescope for about twelve hours.

By 11:00 pm the experimenter had all the equipment ready to observe the hole. The only missing information was the exact coordinates at which the Shuttle would burn the ionosphere and this information would be given in a phone call from Houston at about 11:45 pm.

At about 11:30 pm a technician reparing a phone line damaged by a thunderstorm accidentally turned on a switch that caused a shutdown of all phone communications. The closest phone to the observatory is about half an hour away by car. The atmosphere in the observatory was tense. Some other workers were teasing the technician while he tried to recover the communication lines. They were telling him that due to his blunder the experiment would fail. The experimenter was nervous; the technician was even more nervous.

Sometime around 11:50 p.m. the technician fixed the line, communication with Houston was possible, and the experimenter received the coordinates. The data was collected and everything looked as if it was all right.

I realized afterwards that nothing of what I related here will be known to someone looking at a research paper on this experiment. A lot of the work done by the maintenance employees, the technicians, and the scientists remains hidden and unrecognized by someone just looking at the results. But all this work is important and essential to the progress of research.

Also unnoticed remain the human qualities of all these personnel, which in a given circumstance may affect the outcome of their joint endeavor. In my example, the worker's response of enjoying the technician's misfortune could have impaired his ability to fix the line quickly. In other instances workers were extremely helpful to one another, and better than usual working situations were created. Whenever human beings interact, human qualities will show up, some favorable and some unfavorable, and in the same way that they could affect the result of an experiment they could also have an effect in other fields of work.

# Essay# 50

During my secondary education at The Hill School, in Pottstown, Pennsylvania, I organized a voluntary program to assist the mentally retarded, especially those ignored by their families. Most were middle-aged men suffering from loneliness or depression, and many were given to self-inflicted violence. By arranging surprise parties and picnics, or teaching them songs and games, we gave them companionship and strove to remove their desolation and depression. I have often wondered about the lives of my friends at The Pennhurst House, where they resided. Although I was happy to be able to lead them to see their lives positively through the daily activities we offered, I felt that I was not doing anything really to help cure them. My understanding of their unspoken sufferings made me want to be in a position where I could alleviate the pain in their lives.

My experiences at the Cornell University Medical College reinforced my decision to become a physician. I spent one semester in the Cornell Field Study Program and three summers at the medical college in order to learn about both academic and clinical aspects of medicine. On weekdays, I worked in a cardio-electrophysiology laboratory, using sodium-selective and calcium-selective microelectrodes in order to investigate pharmacological aspects of Digitalis on intracellular sodium and calcium ion activities in cardiac Purkinje fibers. I worked with little supervision and learned to be creative and patient in carrying out the projects. The intellectual challenge and satisfaction that I received, especially after achieving progress, made me seriously consider continuing this learning experience. On weekends, I worked as a volunteer in the emergency room, carrying blood and body fluid samples to the pathology department and transferring emergency patients to their designated rooms. My hospital experiences confirmed my beliefs about what a physician should be in a hospital: As an investigator of diseases, a physician must be competent in his field of medicine; furthermore, as a leader of a healing team, he must know how to lead a group and to communicate well with his fellow workers; but, most importantly, as a counselor, he must be compassionate towards his patients and be willing to guide them. Medicine requires competency, communication, and compassion. Reflecting on the experiences that I had both at the medical research laboratory and the emergency room, I found that I liked what I

would do as a physician, not only to fulfill my daily responsibilities, but also to take up the challenges of solving new and
crucial problems in patient care and medical research.

My undergraduate years have challenged and improved my intellectual creativity, social responsiblity, and personal integrity.
Taking the intitiative to design an independent research course
and a Field Study Program for a semester, I gained much
perspective about the nature of scientific studies. Fulfilling
responsibility as a student representative in the University
Board on Health Service, and in the AIDS Prevention Committee, I learned to educate the community about the importance of
preventive attitude towards health. As a tutor in the Mathe-
matics Department in the College of Arts and Sciences, and as
an orientation counselor, I enjoyed the role of a teacher and
learned to be a more effective communicator. As captain of an
intramural soccer team and as a Junior Varsity Squash player, I
developed not only stamina, but also self-discipline and organi-
zational skills. Taking photography, playing the piano, and
travelling across various cultures, I have broadened myself
and gained much understanding about the global world and the
people.

I appreciate the variety of experiences I have had, not only
because they have prepared me for the diversity I expect to encounter in a medical career, but also because they taught me
how to lead my life; to use my potential for those who need the
medical help. I would like to pursue both clinical and academic
medicine. Each will enrich the other in improving patient care
and medical knowledge. I know that the M.D. degree will not
automatically guarantee my becoming a good physician; self-
education throughout my life is essential. Believing, like Dr.
Bernard Lown, that "those who can see the invisible can do the
impossible," I look forward to using my Cornell University
liberal arts and sciences education as a solid basis for acquiring
the further training necessary to become a competent and caring physician.

# Epilogue

Medicine is not only an applied science, it is also an art, and the art of medicine lies in the healer's insight, empathy, and ability to communicate with the patient effectively. Young physicians must enter medicine compassionate and dedicated to a professional calling.

We stress these essential qualities because, all to often, applicants who could be great physicians get discouraged from applying. If you have a sincere interest in serving the sick, **don't underestimate your fitness for medicine.** A low grade point average or mediocre MCAT scores should not dissuade you from becoming a physician.

Follow the formula we have outlined, have a positive outlook toward medicine and the admissions process, persevere, and you *will* be offered an acceptance to a medical school. Do your best—no one can ask for more. Remember, top-notch applicants with the proper outlook and personality are always in high demand.

**Destiny is not a matter of chance, it's a matter of choice. It's not something to be waited for, it's something to be achieved.**

**—Robert Browning**

The bureaucracy and stress involved in the admissions process may cloud your original goal and diminish your desire. Try not to let yourself get disillusioned and discouraged, and be patient. In time you *will* be practicing medicine, and you *will* be in a position to really help others.

We still recall vividly the hassle of marketing ourselves and the anxiety we felt during the admissions process. Writing the essay, completing applications on time, buying the appropriate suit to project the proper image, sweating during the interview, checking the mailbox several times a day for an acceptance/rejection letter—it's all part of the rites of passage to medicine. Repeatedly, we would ask, "Is it *really* worth it?"

Well, now we can honestly answer, "Yes." There is always something new to learn about disease, patients, and even yourself. Medicine becomes a philosophy that assigns meaning and purpose to our society. Most significant, there is no greater feeling than knowing that every day as a doctor you are able to make a difference in the life of another.

We wish you the best of luck in your career. You have made it this far, and taking the initiative to read this book shows you are heading in the right direction. Have confidence in yourself and your accomplishments, and one day you *will* become a physician!

# About the Authors

**John A. Zebala,** an M.D.-Ph.D. graduate of Cornell University Medical College in New York City, is a resident in pathology at the Univ. of Washington Medical Center in Seattle. He hopes to use molecular approaches to solve basic clinical problems.

**Daniel B. Jones** graduated from Cornell University Medical College and is now a surgical resident at Barnes Hospital in St. Louis. He graduated with an A.B. in Biology & Society from Cornell University. His current research at the Washington University Institute for Minimally Invasive Surgery focuses on applications of advanced technology and the development of new laparoscopic operations.

**Stephanie B. Jones** graduated from Washington University School of Medicine after completing her first two years of medical school at New York University School of Medicine. She received a B.S. in Biochemistry with Honors and Distinction from Cornell University. She is a resident in anesthesiology at Barnes Hospital in St. Louis and is currently expecting her first child (entering medical school in 2015?).

# More Great Books
# from Mustang Publishing

**Working in T.V. News: The Insider's Guide** by Carl Filoreto, with Lynn Setzer. Written by veteran television journalists, this is the most practical and most thorough guide to the T.V. news business available. With complete information on the variety of jobs in a T.V. news department, the hard truth about salaries and hours, advice on creating a résumé tape, a description of an average day in a T.V. news operation, and much more, this book is a must for anyone considering a career in broadcast journalism. *"Should be mandatory reading."*— *Journalism Educator.* **$12.95**

**The Complete Book of Beer Drinking Games** by Griscom, Rand, & Johnston. With over 500,000 copies sold, this book is without a doubt the imbiber's bible! From descriptions of classic beer games like Quarters and Blow Pong to hilarious new contests like Slush Fund and Beer Hunter—plus lots of funny cartoons, essays, and lists—this book remains the party essential. *"The 'Animal House' of literature."*—*Dallas Morning News.* **$8.95**

**Let's Blow thru Europe** by Thomas Neenan & Greg Hancock. The essential guide for the "15-cities-in-14-days" traveler, this is the funniest, most irreverent, and definitely most honest travel guide ever written. With this book, you can blow off the boring museums and minor cathedrals and instead find the great bars, restaurants, and fun stuff in all the major cities of Europe. *"A riot!"*—*The Daily Northwestern (Northwestern U.).* **$10.95**

**Festival Europe! Fairs & Celebrations throughout Europe** by Margaret M. Johnson. What's the best—and least expensive—way to interact with Europeans and their cultures? Attend their myriad festivals, celebrations, fairs, and parades, most of which are free! From the somber Holy Blood Procession in Bruges to the wild Oktoberfest in Munich, this guide will help any traveler have a terrific, festive time in Europe. *"Plenty of good information."*—*Los Angeles Times.* **$10.95**

**Europe on 10 Salads a Day** by Mary Jane & Greg Edwards. A must for the health-conscious traveler! From gourmet Indian cuisine in Spain to terrific pizza in Italy, this book describes over 200 health food and vegetarian restaurants throughout Europe. *"Don't go to Europe without it!"*— *Vegetarian Times.* **$9.95**

**Europe for Free** by Brian Butler. If you're on a tight budget — or if you just love a bargain — this is the book for you! With descriptions of thousands of things to do and see for free all over Europe, you'll save lots of lira, francs, and pfennigs. *"Well-organized and packed with ideas."* — *Modern Maturity.* **$9.95**

*Also in this series:*
**London for Free** by Brian Butler. **$8.95**
**DC for Free** by Brian Butler. **$8.95**
**Hawaii for Free** by Frances Carter. **$8.95**
**The Southwest for Free** by Mary Jane & Greg Edwards. **$8.95**
**Paris for Free (Or Extremely Cheap)** by Mark Beffart. **$8.95**

**Australia: Where the Fun Is** by Goodyear & Skinner. From the best pubs in Sydney to the cheapest motels in Darwin to the greatest hikes in Tasmania, this guide by two recent Yale grads details all the fun stuff Down Under — on and off the beaten path. *"Indispensable"* — *Library Journal.* **$12.95**

---

Mustang books should be available at your local bookstore. If not, send a check or money order for the price of the book, plus $2.00 postage *per book,* to Mustang Publishing, P.O. Box 3004, Memphis, TN 38173 U.S.A.

Allow three weeks for delivery. For rush, one-week delivery, add $3.00 to the total. *International orders:* Please pay in U.S. funds, and add $5.00 to the total for Air Mail.

For a complete catalog of Mustang books, send $1.00 and a stamped, self-addressed, business-size envelope to Catalog Request, Mustang Publishing, P.O. Box 3004, Memphis, TN 38173.

# DARK LORD

## ETERNAL DETENTION

~~This book is dedicated to my mother, Dorothy Thomson~~

Hah, nice try, Thomson, you wormling! This book is actually dedicated to the greatest mind of the 21st century – in this case, myself, Dirk Lloyd!

ORCHARD BOOKS
338 Euston Road, London NW1 3BH
*Orchard Books Australia*
Level 17/207 Kent Street, Sydney, NSW 2000

First published in the UK in 2014 by Orchard Books
ISBN 978 1 40833 025 8

Text © Fabled Lands 2014
Illustrated by Freya Hartas

Dirk's Seal by Russ Nicholson
The right of Jamie Thomson to be identified as the author of this work has been asserted by him in accordance with the Copyright, Designs and Patents Act, 1988.

1 3 5 7 9 10 8 6 4 2
Printed in Great Britain

Orchard Books is a division of Hachette Children's Books, an Hachette UK company.

www.hachette.co.uk

ETERNAL DETENTION

JAMIE THOMSON

ORCHARD

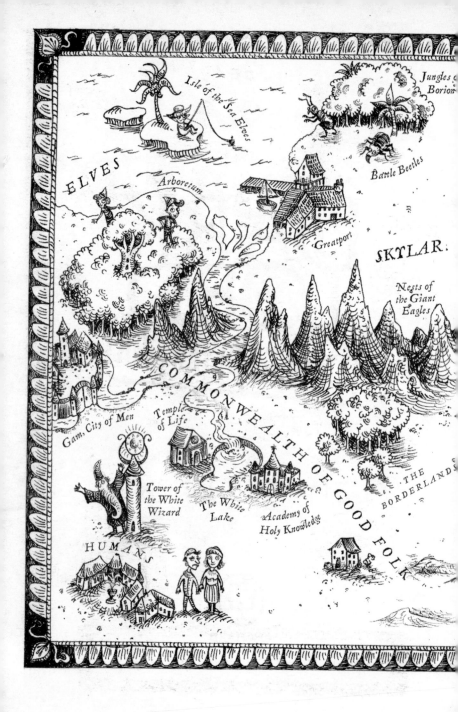

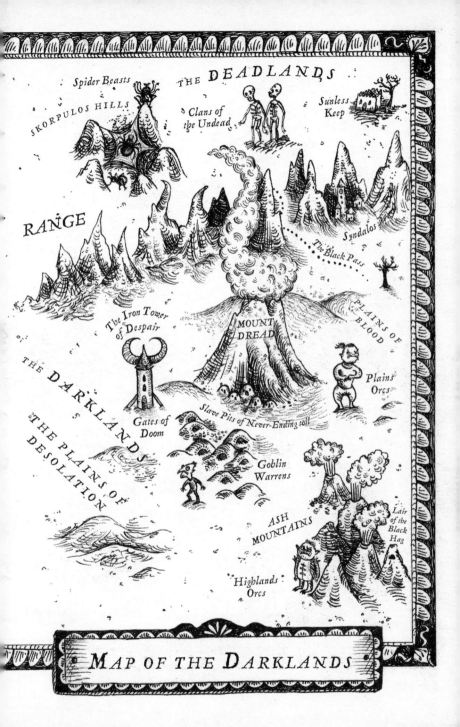

THE **DEADLANDS**

Spider Beasts

SKORPULOS HILLS

Clans of
the Undead

Sunless
Keep

RANGE

Syndalos

The Black Pass

PLAINS OF BLOOD

The Iron Tower
of Despair

MOUNT
DREAD

Plains
Orcs

THE **DARKLANDS**

Gates of
Doom

Slave Pits of Never-Ending toll

THE PLAINS OF
DESOLATION

Goblin
Warrens

ASH
MOUNTAINS

Lair
of the
Black
Hag

Highlands
Orcs

MAP OF THE **DARKLANDS**

# Contents

# A Message from the Dark Lord

For those foolish humans who have not yet read those great works of soaring genius – *Dark Lord: The Teenage Years* and *Dark Lord: A Fiend in Need* – here is a summary of previous events. I, the Dark Lord, was exiled to your pitiful planet by that meddling madman, the White Wizard Hasdruban. To make matters worse, he cursed me into the body of a puny human boy – oh, the indignity! I tried to tell everyone I was the Dark Lord, but, being stupid humans, they all thought I said 'Dirk Lloyd' and that became my name. Being fuss-pot meddlers, these ridiculous humans forced me to go to school, and live with foster parents.

Sigh.

At least I made some friends – or lackeys as I prefer to call them – Sooz and Christopher.

At first, I'd planned to conquer your wretched planet, but soon realised that would be impossible. My legions of Orcs and Goblins were no match for your cunningly constructed tanks, jets and nukes. Instead, I turned my evil genius to the task of getting home to the Darklands. I concocted a nefarious plan, but things didn't turn out as I'd intended and I burned down – no, wait, I mean the cricket pavilion got burned down! Nothing to do with me... Ahem.

My next spell went wrong too, (not my fault, of course!) and instead of propelling me back to the Darklands, it sent my friend Sooz...

Sooz took over my Tower of Despair and ruled in peace and harmony – she says. *Bah*, what a lot of do-gooding nonsense! Anyway, Hasdruban tricked her and imprisoned Sooz in his White Tower. Of course, me and my ~~friend~~ lackey Chris turned the tables on her, and found a way to get to the Darklands. Along the way, Christopher was covered in stinky paste, forced to wear pink underpants and nearly killed, which was funny! Well, I thought so, but Chris...well, whatever. Anyway, we snuck into the the White Tower to rescue Sooz, and I had to cast a very dangerous spell to get her out. It looked like I was going to die so Sooz and Chris had to give me the Essence of Evil, the black goo I'd coughed up when I first fell to your to earth, to save me. It turned me back into a twelve foot tall, hoofed and horned Dark Lord, which was great! But then – how can I put this? I just got more and more...well, *evil*, until finally I lost it completely and locked them both in the Dungeons of Doom. Anyway, Agrash, my Goblin Chancellor, smuggled in a magic crystal which Chris and Sooz used to propel us all (including the monster Gargon and the Paladin Rufino) back to earth. Along the way, I turned back into the boy Dirk, coughing up the Evil Essence once more, which was a relief really, I can tell you. It's quite exhausting being a proper evil Dark Lord... Anyway, we all got home safely. Chris had taken the black, oily Essence and hidden it away, so I couldn't get to it. All seemed well.

Except that the White Wizard had got there before us, taken over the school and made himself the new headmaster, Dr Hasdruban...

Uh oh...

# A Bit of a Squeeze

'AAAaaaarghhhh!' howled Dirk. 'That hurts!'

The bathroom door swept open, and Dirk's foster brother, Christopher, poked his head round the corner, a look of panic on his face. He was blue-eyed and yellow-haired, and would have been rather angelic-looking but for the livid scar that ran down one cheek.

'Are you OK, Dirk?' he asked. Dirk turned to Christopher, a plaintive look on his face.

'Why does it suck so to be a human child?' he said. 'I mean, squeezing spots is such agony!'

'Ohhh!' said Chris. 'Yeah, that hurts, doesn't it? Still, not as bad as having your cheek gouged open by a twelve foot high, horned and hoofed evil Dark Lord, though, eh?'

Dirk turned away, unable to meet Chris's eye. He looked for a moment as if he were going to...well, *apologise*. But Dark Lords never say they are sorry. Instead he scowled at himself in the mirror and said, 'Are you going to upbraid me with this every time we talk, Christopher? I'm not that...thing any more. I'm not like that, it wasn't me!'

'It wasn't me! It wasn't me!' mocked Christopher, fingering his scar. 'That's your excuse for everything, isn't it, true or not!'

Dirk turned and glared at Christopher. 'Do not address me in such tones! I am no petty-minded boy child who must justify himself or face detention. I am the Great Dirk, and you will address me with the proper respect I deserve!'

Christopher raised his eyes. 'Oh, pleeease,' he said, before ducking out of sight and slamming the door.

Dirk turned back and examined the angry face that was looking out at him. Suddenly, instead of a slightly podgy, dark-eyed boy-face in the mirror, Dirk saw a massive, skeletal skull, fanged and horned, like the face of evil itself. But it was fleeting, so fleeting Dirk wasn't sure if it had really happened. Maybe it was all in his mind. He shrugged.

'What's a Dark Lord to do...?' he muttered under

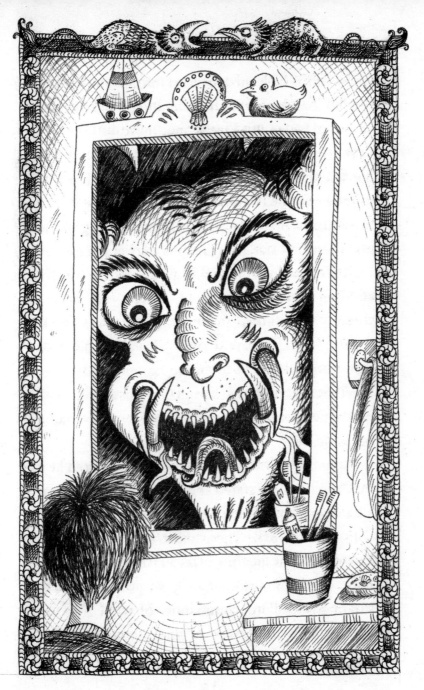

*A typical visit to the bathroom*

his breath as he leaned forward into the mirror and put his hands up to the offending black-headed spot, and began to squeeze once more.

His face knotted up in pain. 'Might be worth considering spot squeezing as a new form of torture in the Dungeons of Doom,' he said to himself.

Suddenly, there was a disgusting plopping sound and the spot burst, spraying pus all over the mirror. Dirk's face wrinkled up in disgust. How vile human children were. But then...

'Wait a minute, that's not pus!' said Dirk. And indeed it wasn't. It was black, and oily and shiny. Astonishingly, it began to move...drawing together...forming itself into a glistening blob of ebony mercury, hanging on the mirror like a parasitical egg.

'Essence of Evil!' whispered Dirk. He stared at it in fascination. He stared and stared. He reached out a hand to the glittering blob of blackness.

Essence of Evil. There must still be some left inside me from the time I was a Dark Lord, thought Dirk. A magnificent, mighty, all-powerful, spell-slinging Dark Lord, commander of armies of Orcs and Goblins and ruler of the Darklands! Dirk paused, hand held out stiffly.

But also selfish, cruel, and heartless. Thoroughly unpleasant, in fact.

Dirk blinked, coming out of his reverie. He didn't want to be that person ever again. The Dark Lord had imprisoned his friends and then almost destroyed them utterly. His friends – or minions, as he preferred to call them, though in his heart of hearts he knew they were really his friends – were all he had in this strange world. And all he had in the Darklands for that matter. He couldn't bear to lose them, not now that he was Dirk Lloyd the human kid. Well, sort of human. His friends had used a special magical crystal – an Anathema Crystal – to bring them all back here to earth, turning Dirk back into a boy and ripping out all the Essence of Evil inside of him. Chris had taken it, and hidden the Essence somewhere so that Dirk could never get his hands on it again. And that's just the way Dirk wanted it; he didn't want to know where it was, in case he got tempted once more. He had made his choice – he would be the boy, Dirk, who had friends, and went to school and lived in modern-day Earth, like everyone else. Well, probably. Maybe he'd go back to the Darklands and live there – he wasn't sure. The important thing was that he'd decided to stay as Dirk. Not any old Dirk, mind you, though. Oh no! He would be the *Great* Dirk. Naturally.

Dirk put a hand to his chin. That was all very well, but what to do with the Essence of Evil? Not much of it, true, not enough to turn anyone totally Evil, but still, it was dangerous stuff. He'd have to store it somewhere, until he could work out what to do with it.

His hand reached for his foster mother's – Mrs Purejoie's – contact lenses case. He emptied the case, throwing the lenses into the bin without a second thought. Gingerly, making sure the Essence of Evil didn't come into contact with his skin, he used the lid to scoop the gelatinous blob into the small contact lens case. He screwed the cap on tightly, slipped it into the pocket of the black, skull-patterned dressing gown that he wore over his Grim Reaper pyjamas and left the bathroom.

He strode purposefully into his room (actually Dirk pretty much strode purposefully everywhere). On the open window ledge sat a gleaming, coal-coloured bird. It cawed at him.

'Ah, Dave, how are you?' said Dirk. Dave the Storm Crow (for that is what it was – an ordinary sparrow that had once tasted a little Essence of Evil and been transformed into a Storm Crow, a red-eyed, black-feathered Harbinger of Doom) hopped up onto his shoulder. Dirk absently stroked its beautiful, shiny black feathers. Well, *he* thought they were beautiful. Not everyone agreed... Actually, no one agreed. Except maybe his friend Sooz, but she was a Goth.

Dirk placed the contact lens case behind a book on the shelf in his room. School next. How unutterably tedious, thought Dirk. Tedious – and very dangerous, now that his arch enemy, the White Wizard Hasdruban, was the headmaster. And today was the day when they'd find out how that was going to go. There was to be a big school assembly, with Hasdruban giving a special talk. Things were going to hot up – eventually there could be only one victor – Hasdruban or Dirk.

Dirk began to put on his school uniform. He had trouble getting his trousers on over the tag around his ankle that the petty and vindictive judge had commanded be put upon him, after he'd been taken to what the humans called 'Court'. A Court of

Justice? Pah! In reality, an absurdly biased-against-evil institution of stuffy old codgers who couldn't be reasoned with in any way whatsoever. Well, ever since Dirk had lost his powers, that is. If he still had all his Darklands magic, then he'd have 'reasoned' with them, oh yes!

Dirk thought back on how he'd been tagged. Sooz had been transported to another world and Dirk and Christopher had gone after her, to that alternate other land, that land of Orcs and Paladins, dragons and eagle riders, a land beyond time and space – the Darklands.

Dirk had once ruled there as the Dark Lord, and fought an aeons-long battle against the Commonwealth of Good Folk and their leaders, the White Wizards, of which there had been many. The three of them had been away for a while, adventuring in the Darklands. Their parents, the police and the school had been frantically searching for them here on earth, assuming the worst.

The three kids had made it safely back but what could they say? That they'd been in another dimension? Where Sooz was the Dark Moon Queen, and Dirk transformed into a huge demon-like Evil

Overlord? No, nobody would have believed it, so they'd made up a story about playing a 'live action role playing game' in a nearby forest, where'd they'd got lost and had to camp out. But even that was scarcely believed.

Naturally, they'd blamed Dirk for most of it, calling him the 'ringleader'. The do-gooding meddlers at the juvenile courts had tagged him and put him on a special curfew and he was going to have to talk to those witless child psychologists, Wings and Randle, too. Still, better than being locked up in an asylum, as he'd have been if he'd told them the truth! And as for the tag...

Well, we'll see about that, thought Dirk.

Once, long ago, he'd been chained up in the dark, deep places of his own land by the forces of so-called righteousness. Chained up for hundreds of years, but still he escaped. Dirk was pretty sure he could find a way around this petty electronic tag. His heart filled with dark purpose, and he said in his most imperious voice, 'I will be free!' He couldn't help himself and he rose to his feet, steepled his hands together in front of his chest (in a gesture he called 'seizing control of the environment') and gave out his best, loudest evil laugh.

'Mwah, hah, hah!'

'Morning, Dirk, you're up then,' said a voice from outside the door. A kind, caring voice, the voice of his foster mother, the Reverend Mrs Purejoie. Dirk sighed.

'Let her not be waiting for me outside the door!' said Dirk to Dave the Storm Crow, who blinked back at him, red eyes glowing. 'She'll want...by the Nine Hells, she'll want cuddles and hugs or something!'

It was time to go to school. No choice. Gingerly, Dirk reached for the handle. Carefully he gripped it...turned...swung the door open – and there in her full holy priestess regalia was Mrs Purejoie, eyes full of love and kindness, arms wide, ready for a morning hug!

'NOOOOOOoooooooooooo!' cried Dirk.

# Whiteshields School Newsletter

## News

### New Headmaster Takes Over

Mr Grousammer, headmaster of the school for fifteen years, has retired on medical grounds. We will miss him, and all the pupils and staff wish him a speedy recovery and a pleasant retirement. He gave so much to the school, including his health. Goodbye, Mr Grousammer!

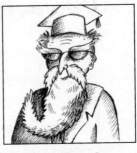

*Dr Hasdruban, the new headmaster*

And welcome to our new headmaster, Dr Hasdruban, recently appointed by the board of governors. Unusually, the board met in secret, but we have been assured that Dr Hasdruban – although unknown to the staff and pupils – has an amazing educational pedigree and we are lucky to have him.

The Chairman of the board of governors, Mr Morris, had this to say, 'Dr Hasdruban... Dr Hasdruban... Dr Hasdruban...' That's all we could get out of him I'm afraid, but anyway, welcome, Dr Hasdruban, to Whiteshields School!

~~November 17th, 2013~~ Rip-out-their-hearts 17th
*Grousammer? Medical grounds? Who are they trying to fool – everyone knows he went mad. As for Hasdruban – well, we shall see!*

# The School Assembly (of Doom)

The new headmaster stepped up to the microphone. He was wearing a white suit, and a white hat and he had a big, bushy silver-white beard. Improbably bushy white eyebrows sprang forth from behind the dark sunglasses he was wearing. In one hand he held a white cane with a curiously carved head on top.

Dirk, standing at the back of the assembly with Sooz and Chris, smiled a half-smile at the sight of his shades. Hasdruban's eyes were as black as night, with no whites at all. That'd freak the humans out if anyone saw them, hence the glasses.

Behind the White Wizard stood another figure, also dressed in white with long white hair and pale, almost translucent skin – Miss Deary, Dirk's old nanny, or the White Witch, as she was known in the

Darklands. And behind her sat several teachers and school governors, seated in chairs.

The Wizard headmaster gingerly tapped the microphone. 'Is this magical device...I mean this... errr...microphone! Is it working?' he said in a deep, commanding voice.

'Yes, sir!' said most of the assembled schoolchildren, who looked on in amazement. Dressed completely in white, with that hairy face and dark glasses? Who was this guy?

'Good. Then I'll begin. I am your new headmaster. You may address me as the White...no, wait. You may address me as "Dr Hasdruban". He paused and looked out over the assembled children. They stared back.

'Today marks the start of a new regime, a new way of doing things! Our creed shall be hard work, discipline and dedication! To what end? Educational attainment, certainly, but that is only a secondary goal!'

The kids blinked up at their new headmaster, confusion written on their faces. What was he on about?

The headmaster's voice grew louder. 'No, our first goal, our most important task, is to root out evil wherever it may be! To crush it utterly! To find it under whatever slimy rock it lies and to destroy it once and for all!'

Some of the teachers shifted uncomfortably in their chairs, eyebrows raised. But not the governors. No, they just stared straight ahead, glassy-eyed. Dirk frowned. Had they been enchanted somehow? Ensorcelled to be the mindless lackeys of their new ruler, the White Wizard?

'And there will be rules! New rules! Rule one: All shall swear fealty and total obedience to the White Wiz...err, I mean to the headmaster!'

Miss Deary put a hand on Hasdruban's shoulder. The Wizard turned to look at her crossly.

'What?' he said. 'Can't you see I'm busy?'

Some of the children began to giggle. The headmaster turned and shouted in commanding tones, 'Silence, wormlings!' Normally, they would have laughed even more at something like that, but Hasdruban did it in such a menacing, threatening manner that they all fell silent.

Miss Deary handed the headmaster a note. She never spoke, you see, and always communicated with written notes. Hasdruban snatched it rudely from her hands and read it swiftly.

Then he looked up. Sighed. And continued, 'Well, all right, there won't be any swearing of oaths of fealty and such, but still, I expect total obedience to my will, or there will be consequences!'

His voice began to rise, and he started to rant madly, 'And when I say consequences, I don't mean your paltry, pitiful punishments like "detention" or "extra homework", I mean death, dismemberment and decapitation, burning, beating and blistering – oh yes, the just desserts for heretics, traitors and the servants of darkness!'

The teachers sat at the back were staring at Hasdruban, jaws agape. The governors, though, smiled indulgently, as if all was well and going to plan. The kids looked back up at him in astonishment too. None of them cracked a joke, no one whispered or made an armpit fart or blew a raspberry. They were too scared.

Miss Deary leant forward again, handing him another note. Hasdruban turned and stared at her. She shook the note under his nose.

'All right, all right,' he said and grabbed it. He read it, then threw it to the ground. He made a face.

'By the Nine Hells!' he barked, shaking his head in frustration. He put his hands on his hips and heaved another sigh. '*Bah!* Well... So then... I was just... joking! Yes, joking, of course there will be no...none of that. However, there will be discipline! Harsh and uncompromising! Detentions will be handed out! Extra homework assigned, to the letter of the law!'

He paused for a moment, to glare menacingly at the assembled children.

'And now, on to Rule Three,' said Hasdruban. 'Informing! All pupils are expected to tell on their fellows, "to dob them in", as you call it. Any wrongdoing, any indiscretion, no matter how minor, must be reported to me! Especially with regard to EVIL! Do you understand me? EVIL must be hunted down and rooted out! EVIL must be destroyed!'

Hasdruban raised his cane and pointed it at the assembled children.

'You know who you are, Evil ones!' he began to shout. 'You know, and I know, and you WILL face the wrath of holy justice!'

Spittle flew from his mouth, causing the kids in the front row to shuffle backwards, setting off a ripple of motion away from the headmaster. Hasdruban

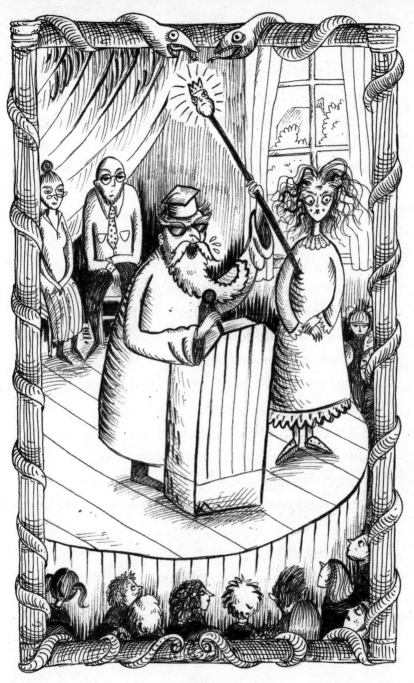

*The headmaster speaks*

paused in his rant and wiped his mouth with a white handkerchief.

'Anyway,' he said, more calmly now. 'To summarise, I am your new headmaster, Dr Hasdruban. I give you Three Rules – Obedience, Discipline and Snitching. Simple enough, eh?'

'Yes, Dr Hasdruban,' said the children meekly.

'Good!' said the headmaster. 'You are dismissed! Off to the dungeons...err...off to class with the lot of you!'

Silently, the astonished children began to file out of the assembly hall, most of them plainly terrified.

Dirk exchanged looks with Sooz and Chris as they shuffled out along with them.

'I'm guessing you're the Evil he's on about,' whispered Chris.

'Do you think?' said Dirk. 'Not just me, though,' he added, 'you two as well.'

'I wonder how that will affect our school reports – *Sorry about being named as an Evil One, Mum!*' said Chris.

'Hah – *Don't worry, Mum, it sounds worse than it is... honest!*' whispered Sooz, grinning.

Trying not to giggle out loud, the three 'evil ones' left the hall.

# Eternal ~~Damnation~~
# Detention

D irk looked up at the clock on the wall. Detention would be over soon. He leaned down and itched his ankle where the tag chafed against his leg and went back to examining the blueprint he was working on – he'd convinced the 'Overseer of Slaves', Grotty Grout (History teacher, bit of a historical relic himself, like a master from a 1950s public school) that it was extra electronics homework. In fact, it was something far more interesting than petty human study.

He looked over at his other companion in detention, Phil Miller, the school bully – he wouldn't even look at Dirk. Tried to keep away from him as much as he could, in fact, after several run ins with Dirk had left him humiliated. Dirk grinned an evil little grin at the memory. Then the bell rang.

'That's it, I hoped you've learned your lesson, boys,' said Mr Grout.

'Yeah, yeah,' muttered Phil Miller, as he hurried out the door, trying to get away from Dirk as quickly as possible. Dirk grinned again. Mr Grout flinched at the sight of it – Dirk's sinister smile had that effect on people.

'Errr...I don't suppose you've learned your lesson, Dirk?' said Mr Grout, stepping towards the door as if he too wanted to make a quick escape.

'Of course not, Grout. Now, get out of my way, I have things to do,' said Dirk commandingly.

Mr Grout looked angry and outraged for a moment and considered giving him another detention – it should be *Mr* Grout, for a start, before you even got to the astonishing insolence of the rest. But then...it was Dirk Lloyd, the most difficult, bright, brilliant, sinister, cunning, uncontrollable kid with an answer for everything he had ever had the misfortune to teach. His shoulders slumped. 'Yes, Dirk, off you go,' he said resignedly.

In any case, thought Dirk to himself, as he waited for old Grout to shuffle out of the way, the lesson was one he had learned a long, long time ago – those with power will inevitably abuse it. After all, he should know. This detention, for instance – it was completely unjust. And not just because he was above all petty rules and should never be subjected to punishment or control, for he was a mighty Dark Lord, but because it actually was unjust, for once. He hadn't done anything wrong (not for want of trying, mind).

No, it wasn't him, it was the headmaster. He'd initiated a campaign of harassment against Dirk. At least it wasn't 'death, dismemberment and decapitation, burning, beating and blistering', thought Dirk with a knowing smile, but still the White Wizard had been putting him in detention every day for a week now. He'd stuck him with extra homework, and special counselling, and extra sport, and remedial classes and whatever else he could throw at Dirk. Worse, the counselling was going to be with those witless fools, Wings and Randle! It was a campaign of spoiling distraction, designed to keep him tied up, so he didn't have time to come up with a strategy or one of his famously complex evil schemes. Maybe it was also designed to break him, to load him with unending tedium. But it wouldn't work, oh no, thought Dirk to himself, he'd survive it, *and* find a way to strike back!

Dirk stepped out of the detention room – and stopped suddenly, for there was his nemesis in the flesh, standing at the end of the corridor! Dr Hasdruban. Next to him stood the deputy head. The White Witch of Holy Vengeance.

They just stood there, staring at him. Dirk folded his arms, raised his head a little, and stared back at them defiantly. The White Witch's tongue flicked from her mouth, like a serpent tasting the air. Dirk grinned his evil grin. The Witch and the Wizard exchanged a look. Hasdruban raised his cane menacingly. Dirk frowned.

But then Mr Grout shuffled out from the detention room. Hasdruban and the Witch turned away, as if they'd just been passing by – wouldn't do for the headmaster to be seen annihilating a pupil with some kind of magical thunderbolt on school grounds, now would it, thought Dirk, chuckling.

Mr Grout shuffled on towards the school exit. Dirk decided it would be prudent to follow him, sticking close to Grout, in case the headmaster and his deputy came back. Having Dirk behind him made Grout a little nervous, of course, so he started glancing back at him from time to time. He could see Dirk doing much the same, though Dirk was checking to see if the Witch and the Wizard were following him too. But to Mr Grout, it seemed like Dirk was checking to see if the coast was clear, probably because he was going to pull some kind of nefarious stunt on Grout, like sticking an 'I'm an idiot' poster on his back, or pinning a long monkey tail to the bottom of his jacket. So Grout began to shuffle forward a little faster. Dirk, wanting to stay close to Grout so that Dr Hasdruban couldn't catch him alone, speeded up too. So did Grout once more, until by the end both of them ended up running out of the school gates as if they were being chased by the devil himself!

Which is what each in their own way actually thought was happening.

Waiting outside the gates were Sooz (dressed in black, of course, with silver jewellery everywhere, wearing chunky Goth boots), and Christopher, still in his school uniform. Both of them stood there staring in amazement at the sight of what looked like Grotty Grout being chased out of the school by Dirk.

Both Dirk and Grout pulled themselves up when they saw Sooz and Chris staring at them in astonishment. Grout and Dirk coughed self-consciously, trying to look normal, as if nothing untoward or strange was going on. Grout took off his jacket, to check the back. Relieved to find nothing wrong, and seeing Dirk strolling over to Sooz and Chris, he hurried away, leaving the three children to their own devices.

'What was that all about?' said Sooz, nodding at the retreating Grout.

'Grout? Oh...errr...nothing, nothing,' said Dirk, glossing over it. He didn't really want to explain that he'd been using Grout as cover to keep himself safe from Hasdruban. All a bit embarrassing, really, for a Dark Lord.

'Nothing? It looked like you were chasing Grotty out of there like a bat out of hell!' said Chris. 'Hilarious!'

'Indeed, perhaps I was in pursuit of the ailing Grout,' said Dirk, warming to the idea. After all, it sounded a lot better than hiding behind his coat tails.

'Really? Why didn't he just put you in

detention?' said Sooz.

'Umm...enough of this, on to more important matters,' said Dirk in his best Dark Lord voice, changing the subject, 'So, how are things in the Forest of Demons?'

When Dirk, Sooz and Christopher had come back to earth, they'd brought with them Rufino, a human Paladin who wore medieval-style armour and carried a sword, and Gargon, a seven foot tall winged demon-like beast, the Dread Lieutenant of the Dark Lord. They were hiding out in the depths of a nearby forest, a forest Dirk had nicknamed 'The Forest of Demons', after Gargon, though its actual name was Willowdown Wood.

'Good, though Rufino is getting restless,' said Chris.

'I guess we'll have to find something for Rufino to do or he'll wander off. What about Gargon?' asked Dirk.

'He's fine,' said Sooz. 'In fact, sitting around doing nothing but hiding seems to suit him. He's been doing a lot of sleeping and lolling about.'

'*Bah*, he was always a lazy Dread Lieutenant,' said Dirk.

'When can you get out there to see them, then? We

need to come up with a plan, find what we can do with them before they get discovered,' said Chris.

'I know, I know,' said Dirk, 'but I have to deal with this tag first. Neutralise it, so I can go somewhere else other than just home and school.'

'Yeah, but how?' said Chris.

'Let's go to my room, and I'll show you,' said Dirk.

As they talked, they ambled round the back of the school, and made their way down Green Lane, passing the allotments. It was a greyish November day, not too cold yet, but still and quiet with a musty dampness in the air. No one was around – or so they thought. A white van came out of nowhere, screaming around the corner towards them. On its sides, the words 'Purify the World' had been painted in blue. It came to a screeching halt and out of the passenger side leaped a figure – Dr Hasdruban!

The three kids pulled up in surprise as Dr Hasdruban stepped towards them, his cane raised high, his other hand curled up in a strange, arcane gesture, his face a maniacal mask of madness!

'Die, Dark Lord, die!' he shrieked, spittle flying from his mouth and dribbling down his long white beard, 'And you too, evil Moon Queen, and your traitorous lackey, the worthless Christopher!' With that, he pointed his cane at them, as if it were a gun.

Reflexively, Dirk raised up his ring hand, the one with the Great Ring, although its powers were as nothing here on earth, and stepped promptly to the side to take cover.

Behind Sooz...

'A f f l i c t u s A n n i h i l a t u s,' screamed Dr Hasdruban as he shook his cane at them.

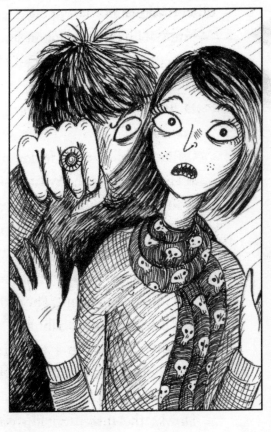

Sooz recoiled, Dirk gritted his teeth, ducking down a bit more, whilst Christopher – Christopher glared at Dirk and stepped in *front* of Sooz, shielding her.

And then – nothing happened. Hasdruban looked

at the cane, puzzled. He shook it once more.

'Die, you hell-spawned creatures of evil, die!' reprised Hasdruban, but still nothing. No blasts of blue lightning or holy fires. Nothing. Then the driver side of the van opened, and out stepped the White Witch. Dr Hasdruban stared at her blankly in confusion. She dashed over and handed him a note. He began to read it.

Dirk smiled, straightening up and stepping out from cover.

'What do you mean it doesn't work? Why not?' said Hasdruban to the White Witch.

'You old fool,' muttered Dirk as he pointed down the road, leading the others on. They began to sneak away, warily skirting the van.

'Really? Only a few minor magics? Are you sure?' said Hasdruban. The White Witch nodded vigorously, furiously scribbling another note.

'Might actually be a human boy? No, I don't believe it, he is the Dark Lord, I tell you!' thundered Hasdruban.

Slowly, the three kept on going, unnoticed for now.

'What are you saying? Of course he deserves

to die!' said Hasdruban faintly, as his voice began to fade. Soon, they'd left the headmaster and the Witch behind.

When they were safely out of earshot, Dirk laughed and said, 'Hah! That witless old Wizard, I would have thought he'd have worked out his magic wasn't going to work here by now!'

Sooz rounded on him. 'Dirk, you used me! You hid behind me! How could you?' she shouted, almost in tears.

Dirk blinked. Chris folded his arms and stared at him, challenging him with his eyes.

'Umm... Errr... No!' Dirk blustered as realisation dawned. 'I...I knew his magic wasn't going to work, of course I did, it was perfectly safe – powerful stuff like that just doesn't work on earth!'

'Really – why'd you hide behind me then, if you knew it was safe?' said Sooz, wiping a little tear from her cheek.

'Ummm... I was hiding something! Keeping it from Hasdruban,' said Dirk.

'Hah, you expect me to believe that!' said Sooz even more angrily. 'Show me then, what was it?'

'What? I...it wasn't an it, it was a...it was a spell, I

was readying a counter-spell, had to keep it hidden and that,' said Dirk, clearly flustered for once.

'Oh, really!' shouted Sooz. 'You just said powerful magic stuff like that doesn't work here, not two seconds ago!'

In the background, up the road a way, two other figures, Hasdruban and the White Witch were engaged in a seemingly similar discussion, waving arms and gesticulating at each other.

Dirk blustered some more, putting on his best Dark Lord voice. 'How dare you question me, puny human girl-child! Don't you know who I am? I don't have to answer to you!'

'Don't try to intimidate me with that, Dirk Lloyd! I'm not just some schoolgirl any more, you know, I've seen off far worse than that!' said Sooz, stamping her foot.

'What about me?' interrupted Christopher who was getting increasingly irritated with the way things were going.

'What do you mean, what about you?' said Sooz and Dirk together.

'Well, you know, I stepped up, didn't I, I stood in front of Sooz, shielding her, not *hiding behind her*,' said Christopher, gesturing towards Dirk. Then he pointed at his own chest, 'Like a hero – a proper hero!' he added loudly.

'Oh yes, you did, that was sweet of you,' said Sooz, stroking his scarred cheek with her hand for a brief second before turning back to Dirk.

'See! Why can't you be more like Christopher?' said Sooz, jabbing her finger at Dirk's forehead.

'Oh, I get it, you want me to be the worthless lackey, so you can take over again!' countered Dirk.

Christopher sighed, as they continued in this vein. The worthless lackey, that's what Hasdruban thought of him, and so did Sooz and Dirk. He might as well not be here. He turned and walked away, leaving Dirk and Sooz arguing in the street. They didn't even notice as his slight form dwindled away in the distance.

*Sooz is rather angry with me. I shouldn't have hidden behind her, I know, but old habits die hard. I mean, what are minions for, after all? Anyway, I felt a little...what's that word that you humans suffer from all the time? Makes you weak and pathetic and blubbersome and all the rest... Ah yes...'guilt'. I actually felt a little guilty. Anyway, I bought her a box of 'Dark Magic' chocolates, which I thought were kind of appropriate. She laughed at that, but still, I don't think she has truly forgiven me.*

*I found this in the paper... Got to do something before it gets out of hand! What if they actually captured Gargon? What would they make of him? Put him in a zoo?*

# The Wendle Herald

## Local News

# The Winged Demon of Sussex

Most of you may recall the so-called sightings of the Surrey Puma or the Beast of Exmoor. Well, now we have a Winged Demon! So far five sightings have been reported of a large, winged beast-like creature, over seven feet tall, stalking Willowdown Wood. Reports say that it resembles some kind of demon out of *Lord of the Rings*! Award-winning psychiatrist Dr Wings said, 'This is a classic example of public fear manifesting itself as hallucination — in medieval times it was demons and gargoyles, in the modern day it's usually been aliens and greys and strange beasts.' Professor Randle, however, said, 'Poppycock, don't listen to that idiot Wings! Probably a big bat and a trick of the light!' Either way, DI Carwen Hughes of the police points out that nobody has been hurt, and there is no need to panic.

# Elecdemonic Tagging

Picture this. A young boy's room. The usual things – bed, a table covered with stuff, chair, large cupboard, shelves with books, Xbox in the corner. All completely normal. Or is it? The bedspread is black with white skulls. The curtains are black – with white skulls. The books aren't your normal kids' books – they're encyclopaedias, books on engineering, advanced electronics, medieval torture techniques, battle tactics, empire building and so on. The table and chair look normal but on closer inspection, the wood has been carved with strange glyphs and symbols. Perched upon the table sits a large black crow with red eyes and feathers like glistening black shadows. It caws, a cry that sounds like the mournful wail of a lonely seagull on a desolate, wind-blasted, corpse-littered shore. Two things lie at its feet – some kind of phone, with little skulls at each corner and bony arms and legs ridging its sides, its opaque, dark surface glowing with a soft shadowy darkness. It is the DarkPhone, built by Dirk using human electronics and necromantic magic so that he could contact Sooz in the Darklands. Beside it is some kind of device that would wrap around a wrist or an ankle, but instead of a strap, it has skeletal claws to grip with, and its central hub is shaped like a small potato-head.

Three kids – Dirk, Christopher and Sooz – were looking at the little scene on the table. Sooz had what looked like a large guitar slung over her back that was almost as big as her. Dirk was playing with the ring on his finger. Sooz glanced over at the ring, a flicker of envy in her eyes. It was the Great Ring of Power, and she had worn it once, wielded its mighty magics like she was born to them, when she'd been Queen in the Darklands. Here on earth, it was powerless. She still wanted it, though, but Dirk had made it clear he wasn't giving it back any time soon. Even though he had once gifted it to her...

Chris fingered the scar on his cheek. 'Is that... some kind of Darktag or something?' he said.

'Yup,' said Dirk. 'Using my superior intellect

and astonishing all-round general greatness, I have replicated your electrical tagging device with a version of my own. Powered by dark magic. Elecdemonic tagging, I call it.'

'Heh, nice,' said Sooz.

'How does it work?' asked Chris.

'Watch,' replied Dirk, and he flicked the little head with a finger. 'On, tiny head, on!'

A pair of little eyes flicked open – causing Chris and Sooz to step back. It began to open its mouth as if to yell. But all that came out was a low buzz. Then it shut its mouth. It opened it wide once more as if yelling, but only that mild buzz came out again. It kept doing that until Dirk flicked the head again. The head twitched as if in irritated annoyance before slumping back into sleep.

'Basically, it yells the same signal at the same frequency as my electronic tag,' said Dirk. 'So when it's on, I can turn my own tag off, and no one will notice anything different. They'll think I'm still here in my room!'

'Cool,' said Chris, 'so now you can get around!'

'Indeed, my puny human friend, I can – I think it is time for me to visit the Forest of Demons, wouldn't you say?' said Dirk.

'We need to get some more supplies too – Gargon doesn't half eat!' said Sooz.

Just then there was a knock on the door. Quickly, Dirk shooed Dave the Storm Crow out of the window, where it hopped onto a little perch Dirk had attached to the outside wall, whilst Christopher and Sooz hid the phone and the tag in a drawer.

'Hello, Dirkikins, it's me, Hilary,' said a voice from outside the door. 'Can I come in please, dear?'

'My name is Dirk, but yes, Mrs Purejoie, you may enter. If you must,' said Dirk, glancing at Chris and raising his eyes at the insufferable '*Dirkikins*'. Christopher did not smile back, which Dirk thought a little odd, but he didn't have time to dwell on it.

The door opened and Mrs Purejoie walked in the room. Tall, thin and blonde, she was wearing the clothes of an Anglican vicar (for that is what she was). To Dirk, it still reminded him of the uniform of the ancient Order of the Assassin Monks of Syndalos, a murderous sect of deadly killers, way back when in the Darklands.

'Hi, Mum,' said Christopher.

'Hello, children,' said Mrs Purejoie. 'Have either of

you seen my contact lenses? They're usually in a little grey case with a cap?'

Dirk blinked guiltily and flicked his eyes to a spot on his bookshelf where he'd hidden the case behind a book. He'd completely forgotten that he'd used her contact lenses case to hide the Essence of Evil. Then he remembered what he'd done with the lenses. What had he been thinking?

Christopher caught his look, and narrowed his eyes at Dirk, with that expression on his face that Dirk recognised so well. It meant, 'What have you been up to now, you devious little freak?'

Dirk gave Chris the Shrug of Innocence, as he called it. Or, more accurately, the Shrug of Feigned Innocence.

'No, I'm afraid not, Mrs Purejoie,' said Dirk. 'Haven't seen them anywhere – but I'll keep an eye out!' He couldn't help himself and added under his breath, 'Your eye – on the table, blinking up at people, heh, heh.'

'Me neither,' said Chris, still staring at Dirk. 'I'll let you know if I see them, Mum,' he said.

'Nor me,' said Sooz, 'Sorry, Hilary.'

'Ah well, I thought as much,' she said. 'I'll check the

fridge, or the tea cupboard. I'm getting so absent-minded these days, I could have put them anywhere! Have a nice day at school, my little chicks.'

"Little chicks?" thought Dirk to himself, raising an eyebrow as Mrs Purejoie left. If only she knew...

'Wait for me downstairs, guys,' said Dirk to Chris and Sooz. 'I've just got to check the... I mean, go to the loo. Cluck cluck!'

With that he hurried off to the bathroom, leaving Chris and Sooz to groan loudly at the chicken joke.

Dirk locked the bathroom door, and began rifling through the bin. 'Ah yes, thank the Dark Gods, no one has emptied the bin yet,' he said to himself. The contact lenses were still there. Carefully, he lifted them out, wrapped them in tissue paper, and hurried off. He would sort the Essence out later, transfer it to something suitable, put the lenses back and put the case in the fridge or something, where Mrs Purejoie would find it and no one would be the wiser.

November 19th, 2013 Rip-out-their-hearts 19th
*Hacked this from the school staff website...*
*Minutes of the Board of Governors...*
*Interesting read!*

WHITESHIELDS SCHOOL
BOARD OF GOVERNORS MEETING
18th November 2014

<u>In attendance</u>
Dr Hasdruban, esteemed headmaster.
Governors: Mr Morris, Mr and Mrs Greene
Teachers: Mrs Batelakes, Mr Grout, Miss Barnes
Stenographer: Miss Deary

<u>1. Apologies</u>
All present apologised to Dr Hasdruban and begged his forgiveness for daring to question his authority in the previous meeting. Dr Hasdruban forgave them all.
<u>Addendum, by order of the headmaster: Forgave them all magnanimously from the goodness of his heart, whilst also reminding them of the penalties for treachery.</u>
Mr Grout pointed out that the word 'treachery' was a bit of an exaggeration and wasn't really appropriate for a school governor's meeting.
Dr Hasdruban pointed out that if Mr Grout didn't like it, he might find that he'd be clapped in irons and hauled off in front of a Conclave of Inquisitors and tried for heresy.
Mr Grout pointed out that Inquisitors didn't exist, and hadn't for hundreds of years. Dr Hasdruban 'pointed out' that that was going to change, and soon.
Mr Grout expressed disbelief. Dr Hasdruban said [comment deleted]
Mr Grout left the room.

## 2. New School Logo
Dr Hasdruban submitted a new design for the school coat of arms.

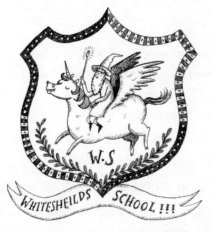

Mrs Batelakes expressed the opinion that such images weren't appropriate for a school
[THIS SECTION DELETED]
Mrs Batelakes left the room.

## 3. Establishment of Conclave of Inquisitors
Dr Hasdruban moved to establish a new board of inquiry to root out EVIL and HERESY in all their forms, wherever they are to be found, especially in the school.
Miss Barnes voted against.
Dr Hasdruban pointed out [comment deleted]
Miss Barnes left the room.
Remaining governors all voted in favour.

# Demons of the Forest

Dirk, Sooz and Christopher sat on a log in a clearing deep inside Willowdown Wood. In front of them stood a seven-foot winged demon from another world, and a tall, lean, fit-looking human. He seemed almost as out of place as the strange seven-foot creature – always looking around in bemusement, a puzzled look on his face. Behind them were two tents, one man-sized, the other much larger. Nearby, a kind of lean-to made out of a tarpaulin on sticks protected a set of drums from the elements. Chris and Sooz had unloaded various supplies earlier as well: bottles of water, blankets, tins of food, camping gas and so on – even a small diesel-powered generator!

The man spoke. 'We can't stay here for ever, Dirk,' he said, gesturing to the tents. 'I mean, it's late autumn now, and when winter comes we will freeze.'

'Gargon hate cold!' said the seven-foot demon.

Dirk put a hand to his chin and stroked it ruminatively. 'I know, I know, but what are we going to do with you?'

'Gargon stands out like a sore thumb, to put it mildly,' said Chris.

'And Rufino – no disrespect, but you're not… Well, you don't come over well in the modern age, but I've got some ideas about that,' said Sooz.

'Yeah, we know about your crazy ideas,' said Dirk. Sooz ignored him. That was odd – she never ignored him! What was going on?

'How's the drumming coming along?' said Sooz, pointing at the drum kit.

'Good,' said Rufino enthusiastically. 'I am glad you brought them, my Dark Lady! I like these modern earth drums, much better than the timbrels, tambours and cowhide drums of home!'

'Even Gargon like sound of Rufino on drums – he pretty good!' ground out Gargon in a voice like crunched up rocks in a blender.

'Rufino may have been a skilled troubadour once, but this is twenty-first century England – your band idea is composed of nuts, Sooz, and lots of them!' said Dirk.

'That's just "nuts", Dirk, not "composed of nuts,"' said Chris, raising his eyebrows.

'Oh, right. Yes, yes of course. You're nuts, Sooz,' said Dirk. 'Nuts!'

'Thanks for your support, Dirk – mind you, that's what I've come to expect from you these days,' said Sooz waspishly. Dirk frowned, silenced for once. Christopher gave him a mocking half smile which puzzled Dirk even more.

'Anyway,' continued Sooz, 'I've brought you this, Gargon,' and she handed him the rather large guitar she'd been carrying on her back. 'It's a special big guitar for big handed people. I reckon those talons of yours will be like a handful of plectrums, and you'll make a great lead guitarist!'

Gargon looked at his enormous taloned hands. 'Plec...plec what?' he gravelled.

'Don't worry about that now,' said Sooz, 'just take the guitar and play with it. Here's a book too, on teaching yourself guitar.'

'Hah, hah!' laughed Dirk, 'It's Gargon, for evilness's sake – he can't even read, let alone learn to play the guitar!'

Gargon blinked in embarrassment. He hated people knowing he couldn't read.

'Well, we'll see about that, Dirk Lloyd,' said Sooz huffily. 'I think Gargon has hidden musical talents!' She turned to Gargon, and took him by the hand. 'Don't you, my dear old Gargie?' she said.

Gargon looked down at Sooz affectionately, an expression quite out of place with his overall demeanour – i.e. winged, taloned, scaled and fanged.

'Gargon try, my Queen, Gargon try his best!' he grated.

'Oh please, this is ridiculous,' said Dirk. 'And how'd you guys get all these supplies and the instruments and that over there, that generator, by the Nine Hells?'

Sooz and Chris exchanged a look.

'Gold,' said Chris.

'Gold? What do you mean, gold?' said an astonished Dirk.

'When we came back from the Darklands we both had a few gold coins in our pockets – you know, gold Dirks.' (When Dirk had been in Dark Lord form, ruling the Darklands, he had introduced coinage – Gold Dirks, Silver Soozes and Copper Christophers).

'Worth quite a bit over here,' said Chris.

'Oh, I see, and when were you going to tell me about this?' said Dirk, a little annoyed.

'We...we knew you wouldn't want to spend the money on...well, musical instruments and stuff,' said Sooz.

'You're right there! What a waste. Weapons! That's what we need, weapons – tanks, even! To fight the headmaster.'

'All very well, Dirk, but it's England. You can't buy weapons,' said Sooz.

'Especially when you're kids,' added Chris laughing, 'and especially not tanks!'

Dirk folded his arms. Crashing into the headmaster's study in a tank would have been so cool. But they were right, of course.

'Pah, enough of this,' said Dirk. 'I'll keep on working on the only sensible option – getting them back to the Darklands. Now, let's go, guys, we'll come back with more supplies later!'

'You go if you like, I'm staying here to teach Gargon some basic chords,' said Sooz.

'Me too,' said Chris.

Dirk stood there for a moment. Didn't they want to hang out with him anymore or something? He felt a twinge of hurt and sadness, but then a quiet anger rose up within him. They'd been off with him ever since that business with Hasdruban in a van. Well, so be it. He'd been alone and friendless for a thousand years or more before he'd met these two, he could handle being alone again! He didn't need them, they were worthless humans, anyway. In any case, he needed to get back and sort out the lens situation, a task best undertaken alone.

With that, he turned and headed out of the clearing. He followed the trail they had created through the woods – he'd used Orcish symbols painted in black on the trees to mark the way. No ordinary human would ever understand them, but his friends could. His minions, rather, of course. Disobedient minions, that is. Soon he came to the edge of the wood, and began to cross the farmer's field that led to the bridge at the edge of Whiteshields town and then on towards the bus stop for home.

In a nearby van, a figure in white watched the boy as he trudged up the low hill into town...

~~November 20th, 2013~~ Rip-out-their-hearts 20th

*Out of boredom and disgust at the trite mundanity of the Whiteshields School newsletter, I have decided to create my own little newspaper type thing which I will distribute around the school. I have decided to call it the* Dark Times. *Here's a sample.*

# THE DARK TIMES

Issue One          Price: 5 Copper Christophers

'There are two types of humans – my lackeys, lickspittles and slaves, and those who will soon be my lackeys, lickspittles and slaves.'
Dirk Lloyd

## Today's Horrorscope

~~Scorpio (Deathsting)~~ – Today, a giant scorpion will rise up out of the earth and sting you to death! Mwah, hah, hah! Better stay in.

*Aries (Scaries)* – Today, an enormous comet will fall out of the sky to crush you utterly! Better stay in, if I were you.

*Gemini (One-Two-Many)* – A while back, a mad scientist cloned you. Today, that clone will turn up and kill you, laughing as it does so. Better stay in, I think.

*Leo (Kittenkill)* – If you go out, you will be eaten by wild animals. No, really. Best stay in, I think.

*Libra (Wishwashy)* – Most of your friends have finally realised what a wretch you really are, and they've decided to kill you. Better stay at home, and hope your family aren't in on it too.

## Letters with the Aunt of Agony

Dear Aunt of Agony,

My parents are causing me problems at the moment, I really don't think they understand me. What shall I do?

Yours,

Laura Wibblebottom

*Dear Laura,*
*You need a potion of mind control. Put it in their tea, and they will be as docile as cows, obeying your every command, and doing whatever you tell them to do.*
*Yours Sneeringly,*
*The Aunt of Agony*
*PS By the way, don't let anyone find out what you've done, especially the police.*


Dear Aunt of Agony,
I like animals, but my brother has a pet tarantula. It keeps escaping and hiding in my bed. Well, that's what my brother says, I reckon he puts it there. Anyway, it's harmless, but frightens me so much I can't sleep, as I'm worried it might turn up at any time. What should I do?
Yours,
Sarah Snailweed


*Dear Sarah,*
*Oh my, what an opportunity! Take the spider, hide it in your neighbour's cupboard, feed it up with a massive dose of radioactive growth*

*hormones, and sit back and watch the carnage.*
*Mwah, hah, hah!*
*Yours Sneeringly,*
*The Aunt of Agony*

This issue of the *Dark Times* brought to you by
the Great Dirk!

Yours Unfaithfully,

*I, the Dark Lord, Master of the Legions of Dread and Sorcerer*

*Supreme, the World Burner, the Dark One, Master of the Nine*

*Hells, the Lord of Darkness and the Lloyd of Dirkness, his Imperial*

*Darkness and his Imperial Dirkness, Dirk the Magnificent, make*

*this missive my own with this seal, on this date the 20th of Rip-out-*

*their-hearts, Year of the Dark Lord One, in the Reign of Iron and*

*Shadows. Well, the Reign hasn't officially begun, not quite yet, but*

*soon, oh yes, soon. Just as soon as I get out of detention.*

# Dark Visions

Dirk and Christopher sat around the breakfast table, waiting for Mr and Mrs Purejoie to join them. Christopher was staring at the table. Dirk, who'd been having an imaginary fight between the pepper pot as the Dark Lord, and the salt cellar as the White Wizard, put down the Holy Sword (knife) and the Evil Trident of Utterly Destroying White Wizards (fork) with an irritated flourish.

'What's the matter with you, Christopher?' said Dirk. 'You're moping around like a Goblin in a cage!'

'Nothing,' said Chris morosely.

'What do you mean, nothing? How can it be nothing? Look at you!' said Dirk.

Chris just shrugged disconsolately, and began fingering the scar on his cheek, his mind elsewhere, brooding.

Dirk sighed. What was it with people? These

humans and their curious moods. Up, down, sideways. It wasn't much fun hanging out with Christopher when he was like this. He wouldn't play any computer games or anything!

Dirk frowned. He'd have to snap him out of this mood, if only so he could win a few games of *Fantasy Wars* or that *Blood of Darkness* game. He hadn't crushed a puny human for ages, and Chris was always good for that!

Dirk tied his white napkin around his chin, pretending it was a beard, and said, 'Die, Dark Lord, die!' in a passable imitation of the headmaster, Hasdruban. 'And after you're dead, you're going into detention for a month!'

At that, Chris raised a wry smile, and made a tiny laughing sound. Dirk, encouraged by his comedic impersonation, added, 'And then I shall destroy your worthless lackey, Christopher, too!'

But Chris didn't laugh at that. In fact, he just glared at Dirk angrily. And then his face fell, and he turned back to examining the table.

'What! What did I say?' said a bemused Dirk.

Mrs Purejoie came into the room.

'These contacts seem a little dark, as if they were

sunglasses or something. I found them in the fridge – could the cold darken them up? Is that possible?' she said in puzzled tones.

'That doesn't seem likely,' said Dirk, but inside he was thinking furiously. Darkened? He'd put her lenses back in the case that had held some of the Essence of Evil. He'd cleaned the case out as thoroughly as he could but still – it clung to things like glue. Could her lenses have been contaminated with Essence of Evil somehow? Could it affect Mrs Purejoie in some way? He began to stare at her avidly. This could be interesting!

'What do you think, Christopher, my darling?' she said.

Chris shook his head. 'Doubt it,' he said tersely.

Mrs Purejoie sat down, and then Mr Purejoie came in bearing breakfast for the family. He was a red-haired, ruddy faced man with gentle blue eyes – a GP, in fact. He didn't think the cold would darken Mrs Purejoie's lenses either. After a short prayer (Dirk mumbled his own version under his breath – which usually involved adding the word Dark to any instances of 'Lord' and so on), the family tucked into eggs on toast.

Before Dirk had taken a mouthful, something odd happened. Mrs Purejoie leaned back. 'What... what's that...?' she said in astounded tones. Everyone followed her gaze. She was staring at...well, staring at the corner of the room.

Suddenly she screamed!

'What is it, dear, what is it?' said Dr Purejoie as he leaped up and dashed to her side. Christopher was open-mouthed with shock. His parents never did anything odd or out of the ordinary and they certainly didn't have hallucinations like they'd been taking drugs or something!

'Mum, are you all right? Mum?' he said in worried tones.

'It's a terrible blackness, a desolate... I can see... what...how?' she stuttered, staring in horror at the corner of the room.

'Don't worry, sweetheart, we're here!' said Dr Purejoie, holding her hand, as he tried to work out what was happening to her.

'What can you see?' said Dirk.

'I can see...a tall...a tall black tower...in the middle of...a desolate land...and there are little creatures... ugly little capering things – OHHH, it's awful!'

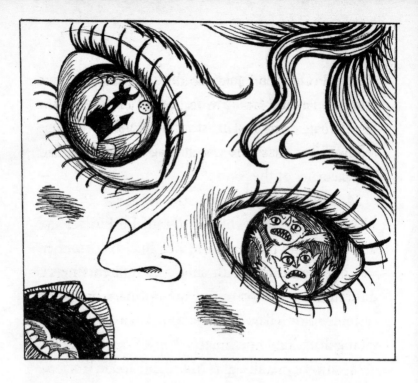

she said. Mrs Purejoie began plucking at her eyes, pulling out her contact lenses. 'It's these contacts... they're evil! EVIL, I tell you!' she said, as she threw them onto the floor.

Everyone stared at her in amazement. Then Chris turned to Dirk, a suspicious look on his face. Dirk gave him the Shrug of Feigned Innocence. Chris narrowed his eyes, unconvinced.

'Now, dear,' said Dr Purejoie, 'I don't think the lenses can be evil, can they? Maybe they got coated in something, and it's distorted your vision.'

Mrs Purejoie blinked rapidly. 'Yes, yes, I'm sure that's it, Doctor Jack. I'm feeling much better now that I've taken them out.'

'Yeah, just dirty lenses,' said Dirk as if nothing had happened.

He put a hand to his chin, staring at Mrs Purejoie like she was a rat in a lab. It sounded like she'd had a vision of the Darklands. Maybe his Iron Tower, in fact, the Iron Tower of Despair. And little creatures... could they be his Goblin servitors? Interesting!

Breakfast continued with the usual inane chit-chat about petty human concerns of day to day life that Dirk blanked out as he considered what had just happened. It had given him some ideas.

Afterwards, Dirk and Chris set off to school. It was a ten minute walk, one they did every day.

'So,' said Chris, 'What have you been up to?'

'Me? Nothing, nothing at all, what do you mean?' said Dirk.

'Don't give me that – you nicked her lenses didn't you? What did you do to them?' demanded Christopher.

'Eh? Nothing, nothing at all!' spluttered Dirk.

'Yeah, right. She's my mum you know, you can't

just experiment on her whenever you like!' said Chris angrily.

'And mine too, by the way! Foster mum, sure, but still,' said Dirk.

'You what? You've never cared about anything like that before – that makes me even more suspicious!'

'Oh come on, I'm not that bad, I wouldn't, I mean I didn't! I didn't do anything, it wasn't me!' said Dirk rather squirmingly.

Chris stopped. So did Dirk. Chris frowned, fingering his scar. 'Hold on a minute, what do you mean, it wasn't you? What wasn't you?'

Dirk raised his eyes. 'Well, it wasn't me – on purpose, that is.'

'Uh huh,' said Chris, 'Now we're getting somewhere!'

Dirk sighed. 'That spot, you know, that hurt so much...' he said.

'Yeah?' said Chris.

'Well, it was like...a Dark Lord spot, kind of thing,' said Dirk.

'What do you mean, "dark lord spot"?' said Chris.

'Umm...instead of pus, it was...a bit of...a bit of Essence of Evil,' said Dirk hesitantly.

'What?' said Chris, aghast. 'I thought it all came out when you fell to earth the last time, with the Anathema Crystal in the Dungeons of the Iron Tower! I scooped it all up when we got back.'

'And hid it, I know, hid it away from me, as we all agreed, I know, I know,' said Dirk.

'If this is some kind of trick to get me to tell you where I hid it, it's not going to work, Dirk! We can't let you anywhere near the stuff, not after what happened last time,' said Chris.

'I know! And I agree, don't tell me. But there must have a been a little left inside me this time. And it bubbled up to the surface as it were. I squeezed it out, and then...well, I had to put it in something, didn't I?' said Dirk.

'Ahhh, now I get it,' said Chris. 'So you put some Essence of Evil into my mum's contact lenses case, and hid it in your room.'

Dirk nodded shamefully. Well, almost shamefully.

'You total numpty, Dirk, that stuff's really dangerous, how could you?' said Chris.

'I just wasn't thinking...' said Dirk. Chris shook his head despairingly.

'I tried to fix it,' continued Dirk. 'Cleaned out her

71

case – but you know what that stuff is like, some of it got must have got into her lenses, gave her those weird visions – but that's all, no harm done, just a one-time freaky vision!'

'As far as we know,' said Chris. Still, it did sound like no permanent harm had been done – she'd be able to get clean replacement lenses easily enough, after all, and the contaminated ones had been disposed of.

'Not all bad, though,' said Dirk, 'As it's given me an idea – I reckon she was seeing into the Darklands, maybe I can try something similar, see what's going on there, maybe even get a message through or something.'

'Whoa,' said Chris, 'It's dangerous stuff, especially for you. I think you should just hand it over to me, and I'll hide it with the rest.'

'No, no, I need to try this, Chris – it might lead to a new way to reach the Darklands. We can send Gargon and Rufino back, maybe even Hasdruban.'

Chris was unconvinced. 'Really? Seems like a long shot if you ask me. Are you sure the Essence isn't making you think weird?' he said.

'No, no, there really isn't that much of it. It doesn't

feel like...you know, like it's taking you over and that. But you're right, it is a long shot, but long shots are all we've got at the moment,' said Dirk.

Chris had to agree with that. 'Well, it's your call, I guess.' After a moment, he added sarcastically, 'After all, I'm just a worthless lackey, right?'

'All the more reason why you shouldn't have called me a numpty, by the way! I would have thought you'd have learned your lesson after the last time you tried that,' said Dirk imperiously.

Christopher scowled angrily. Dirk, of course, simply strode on, oblivious, declaiming his genius, and how people should show him more respect, that he was a great Dark Lord, and how those who insulted him often ended up wearing pink underpants and getting covered in stinky goo.

Chris sighed. But then, nearby, he noticed a middle-aged man in walking boots, outdoor clothes and a backpack, poring over a map. He heard Dirk's loud claims, and raised a surprised eyebrow. His face was so astonished, Chris couldn't help himself and laughed out loud.

'What?' said Dirk. But then the rambler stepped forward.

'Actually, lads, can you help me? I think I'm a bit lost. How do I get to St Mary's Church, the one with the famous stained glass windows? Should be near here,' said the man.

'Of course,' said Dirk. 'Head down the road, turn right, go on a hundred yards, turn left into Castellani Road, and there it is.'

'Oh, right, thanks!' said the man, and off he went.

Dirk and Chris continued on. After a few moments, Chris pulled up short and said, 'Hold on, that was totally wrong – you've sent him in the opposite direction to the church!'

Dirk stopped. 'Oh yeah, so I did!' he said, a look of surprise on his face.

'But why?' said Chris.

Dirk shrugged. 'Dark Lord, I guess. Sometimes I just can't help myself.'

# *Shadowshades*

That evening, after the inevitable detention, Dirk returned to his room and set to work. He reached for a small tin, a pirate tin he'd found in Chris's room with a skull and crossbones on the lid. He'd hidden it behind a book called, *How to Conquer the Earth*. A much read book, by the look of it. Dirk took the tin down, and gingerly opened it. Inside was a congealed blob of black stuff – Essence of Evil. Mrs Purejoie's contact lenses had obviously been contaminated with it, enabling her to see into the Darklands.

Possibly. Dirk was going to find out whether that was true or not.

He reached for a pair of plastic glasses he'd got cheaply from an optician, with the lowest prescription setting you could get. Carefully, he coated the lenses with a thin layer of Essence of

Evil. He watched, fascinated, as it seemed to soak into the glass, giving it a shadowy, greyish sheen. Gingerly, he raised them up and put them on. Everything went kind of grey. And quiet.

Then something appeared in the air in the middle of the room! A tiny black spot, shimmering like a black strobe. It began to grow and widen.

Dirk sat back, gripping the arms of his chair, transfixed. It grew bigger and bigger, until it was the size of large window. Through the black hole shapes began to appear on the other side – a hill, a tall tower... Could it be? Yes, it was the Iron Tower of Despair! Dirk concentrated and the vision moved in closer and closer. He could see the Gates of Doom and the annoying iron gargoyle heads that would never shut up. A couple of heads actually looked straight up at him, as if they could sense something was spying on them. Dirk willed the vision on, into the Tower, but he could not pass through the Gates of Doom. Of course, they were shielded with protective magics. He should have known, he'd put them there centuries ago. But then the great gates began to grind open.

'Hail to the Regent Agrash, and General Skabber,

Keeper of the Tower whilst the Dark Lord and his Lady are in Exile,' screamed several of the gargoyle heads, and out walked Agrash Snotripper the Goblin, and Skabber Stormfart, the Orc Captain. Or General now, it seemed.

Dirk, excited by the sight of them, leaned forward and yelled, 'Agrash, it's me, Dirk, the Dark Lord!!!' but they couldn't hear him. They just walked on, talking to each other in low tones.

'No, we mustn't provoke them, Skabber,' Agrash was saying, wiping the end of his improbably long nose with a stained handkerchief. 'A raid is a really bad idea!'

'Yeah, but the White Wiz ain't at home! Now's the time to give 'em a bloody nose,' said Skabber, itching an armpit with a warty, black-nailed hand. Well, more like a claw really.

'We're still too weak, and we've got a kind of wary peace without the Dark Lord and the White Wizard here to stir things up – let's not upset the boat, Skabber,' said the Goblin.

The Orc frowned. 'What boat?' he said.

They walked on. Desperately, Dirk leaped to his feet, and tried to step through the hole, but it wouldn't let him. He threw himself at the dark window, but all he did was bounce off to crash onto the floor in a heap, having bruised his shoulder. What were they thinking? Keep the peace? The fools! Now was their chance to storm the White Wizard's stronghold!

There was a sudden knock on the door. 'Are you all right, dear?' said a voice from outside his room. Mrs Purejoie, on the prowl!

'I'm fine,' said Dirk, 'everything's fine,' as he quickly ripped the glasses off his face. There was a popping sound and the dark window disappeared in a flash. Mrs Purejoie stuck her head around the door.

Dirk was sitting in his chair, one hand behind his back, hiding the glasses. Mrs Purejoie stared at him for a moment, wondering what he was up to. Probably best not to ask, she thought.

'All right then – time for bed anyway. Pyjamas and clean teeth!' she said, smiling at him sweetly.

Dirk raised his eyes. One minute he was gazing at the Iron Tower of Despair where his Goblin Chancellor and the Captain of his Orcish hordes were discussing battle strategy, the next he had to

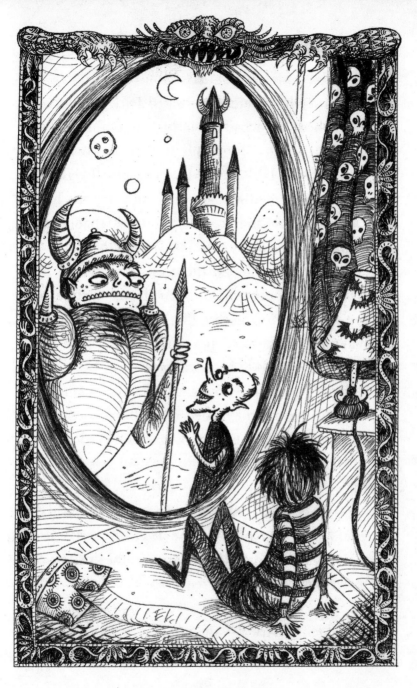

*Window shopping, Dirk style*

clean his teeth and put his pyjamas on.

Half an hour later, an excited Dirk was tucked up in bed. He'd had to endure a goodnight kiss and a hug, but that ghastly torture was over. For now, anyway. Dirk reached for his special glasses – 'dark glasses' had a whole new meaning for him! Or maybe he should call them his shades. Or Moonglasses? No, Shades. His Shadowshades.

Carefully he slipped them on. A vision of the Darklands appeared, his Iron Tower casting an ominous shadow across the plain as the sun set behind it. Dirk stared at it avidly. There must be a way of using this to his advantage.

Dave the Storm Crow gave a low caw as it flew into the room and landed on his shoulder. Dirk absently petted the glistening black bird, as he considered the scene before him. All was quiet in the Darklands.

Dave hopped onto the window into another world, and perched on the ledge between this world and that. It sat there staring at the great black tower with its glowing red eyes. It cawed as if in recognition.

Suddenly Dirk sat up in shocked amazement.

How could Dave perch there? There shouldn't be a 'ledge', nothing could pass through that hole, only sight and sound, surely – and one way only at that. Dirk darted forward for a closer look. Yes, Dave was halfway into the Darklands! Dirk reached forward but he couldn't grab onto the 'ledge'. For him there was no physical window, but it seemed there was for Dave the Storm Crow.

Of course, thought Dirk to himself. Dave was a Storm Crow – a Harbinger of Doom. And a harbinger was a kind of messenger or herald. It made sense that the Harbinger of Doom could travel between the planes much more easily than a human, or even a Dark Lord, for that was what Storm Crows were for. Dirk began thinking furiously. He could write a message to the Darklands, tell them he was alive and well, and that they should hold the fort whilst he worked out how he was going to get Gargon and Rufino home, and whether he should go with them or not. He could strap it to Dave's leg, just like those messenger pigeons the humans used to use. Instruct Dave to take it to Agrash!

'YESSSS!' shouted Dirk, and he stood up, put his fingers together and laughed out loud.

'MWAH, HAH, HAH!!!'

'Oh, do be quiet and go to sleep, Dirk, really!' said Mrs Purejoie sharply from outside his room.

# *Psycho Fools*

The next day at school was an exceptionally dull day of interminable lessons, like wading through a treacle-sludge of liquid boredom. Last night he'd sent Dave to the Darklands with a message written on paper. He'd had to strap it to Dave's leg with a rubber band – hopefully it got through OK. Dave had not returned yet – perhaps it would some time today but Dirk wouldn't know until he'd got back to his room. With luck, Dave would be there, waiting for him. Or maybe Dave could only return when Dirk was wearing the Shadowshades.

All he had to do was get through the rest of the day at school to find out.

Luckily, he didn't have detention tonight, which was a surprise, so he hurried home after school. He was all alone – Sooz and Chris were heading off together to the forest as usual, to teach Gargon and

Rufino how to play drum and fish. No wait, drum and...what was it? Some kind of fish, he was sure of it! Oh yes – bass, that was it. Drum and sea bass. No, that wasn't it. He couldn't remember rightly – some kind or other of pitiful human music. Whatever it was, they were misguided fools. Gargon was the result of an unholy union 'twixt a Demon Lord and a Lich Queen – neither of which were noted for their musical talent, to put it mildly. Rufino was a sworn Paladin, a warrior through and through. There was virtually zero chance that they could be modern earth musicians, it was ridiculous. And because of it all, he hardly saw Sooz or Chris. It was almost as if they were deliberately avoiding him. Not that he cared, of course, they could do what they liked. He frowned. He could feel his eyes filling up with... water, it was just water. Not tears. Dark Lords don't cry! Must be some reaction to exhaust fumes or dust particles or something. Anyway, he had to get to his room, find out what was what. He wiped his eyes, opened up the door, called a brief 'It's me!' to any Purejoies in the house, and ran up the stairs.

He rushed into his room – and there was Dave the Storm Crow, sitting on the perch just outside the window! Dave cawed a greeting, a sweet sound to Dirk's ears, like a lost soul in hell. There was something strapped to the black bird's leg – a little bottle with a message. Dirk reached for it...

...and there was a sudden knock on the door.

'Noooo!' spat Dirk angrily.

Whoever it was knocked again, loudly.

'Hello Dirk, it's me, Miss Cloy,' said a voice from outside the door. Dirk raised his eyes. He'd once thought of Miss Cloy as the Commander of some kind of elite human special ops unit called the Social Services Legion. In fact, she was just a Social Worker. An annoying, meddling, interfering, do-gooding social worker. Dirk clenched his fists. And let out his anger, along with a long sigh. He composed himself, and went over to the door.

'What is it?' he said in his cutest little boy voice, as he opened the door and smiled sweetly up at Miss Cloy.

Miss Cloy took an involuntary step backwards. Dirk didn't realise that what he thought of as his 'sweet smile' was no different from his normal smile, which most people called his 'Hannibal Lector' grin. And as for his cute voice – that sounded like a child possessed by the devil in a horror film.

Miss Cloy stared at Dirk for a second or two. 'I'd forgotten...' was all she could get out.

Dirk made a face. He hadn't got time for this. 'Well, what is it, puny mortal?' he said imperiously, giving up all pretence of childlike sweetness.

Miss Cloy pulled herself together. 'I've come to take you to your counselling therapy session, Dirk.'

'Counselling! Now?' said Dirk, surprised.

'Yes, with Dr Wings and Professor Randle. You've been told about it. Several times. Your parents got a letter, so did you.'

Dirk blinked at her. 'Ah yes, I vaguely recall some such nonsense,' he said. 'But why are you here?'

'Well, because of your curfew tag. You're not supposed to go anywhere but school and home. Except when accompanied by your designated adult. That's me!' said Mrs Cloy.

'By the Nine Hells, how insufferably tedious,' said Dirk rudely.

'Oh come now, Dirk, it'll be like old times,' said Mrs Cloy breezily, trying to make the best of it, and taking him by the arm.

'How dare you lay your hands on the Great Dirk!'

said Dirk unthinkingly. 'Unhand me this instant, upstart human female!'

Miss Cloy blinked at him in astonishment. Then she let go, lifting her hand away theatrically. 'All right, all right! You haven't changed then, have you, Dirk?'

Actually, he had changed quite a bit, thought Dirk, but he didn't know how to explain it or even where to begin, so he just shrugged.

Miss Cloy sighed. 'Well, we have to go, and that's that,' she said.

Dirk made a face. There was no way out. 'So be it,' he said. 'Come on then, let's get it over with, Miss Cloy, as quick as possible!'

Miss Cloy led him to her car – a VW Beetle, which Dirk had once thought of as a kind of battle chariot, similar to the Battle Beetles of Borion he had once bred for his armies back home. In fact, it was just a car – he'd got used to those by now, as they were all over the place here on earth. Though for the life of him, Dirk couldn't work out why they didn't put rams on the front, scythes on the wheels, with added rocket launchers and machine guns. Maybe even a flamethrower on the back to deal with tailgaters.

That would make driving fun!

Burn, tailgater, burn! Mwah, hah, hah! thought Dirk to himself – but it wasn't entirely to himself. He'd 'Mwah, hah, hahed' out loud, and Miss Cloy was looking at him oddly.

'Umm, sorry, I was just consigning other drivers to a fiery death...errr... I mean, the flamethrower... No! I mean...oh, what's the use?' said Dirk.

Miss Cloy shifted uncomfortably in her seat. 'Sounds like you *need* therapy, young man,' she said.

Hah, you have no idea! replied Dirk in his mind. No point in saying it out loud – she would never understand. Well, unless he took her to the Darklands. Heh! Yeah, that would be fun! He stared at Miss Cloy, grinning as he imagined her meeting Rak Rak the Nightgaunt, with Dirk as the Dark Lord sitting on the Throne of Skulls, Agrash with his snot-tap nose, and Skabber and a horde of orcs kneeling before him.

'Stop staring at me. And stop smiling like that, it's really creepy!' said Miss Cloy, clearly rather disturbed.

'Sorry, sorry,' said Dirk, with a chuckle. He turned away to watch the road.

After a short drive, during which Miss Cloy drove rather faster than she should have, Dirk found himself sitting in the waiting room of Dr Wings and Professor Randle's office. Miss Cloy checked her watch. They were early. She got up.

'Back in a moment, Dirk,' she said, and left the room. Dirk contemplated making a run for it, but decided against it. They'd only bring him back again another time. The door to Wings and Randle's office opened and out stepped...Mr Grousammer, the old headmaster! His face was craggy and drawn looking, his suit a little shabby, the tie askew. The oddest thing were his cheeks and chin. Quite thoroughly clean-shaven, but rather red and raw, as if he were suffering from some kind of rash.

Grousammer paused and stared at Dirk. And stared. His eyes flicked to Dirk's left arm, and widened in horror.

Dirk gave him one of his famous grins. The old headmaster raised an enfeebled hand as if in warding, gave a plaintive cry of distress and ran out of the room as fast as he could.

'Wow, wasn't expecting that,' said Dirk to himself. Then he noticed the door was slightly ajar. Quickly

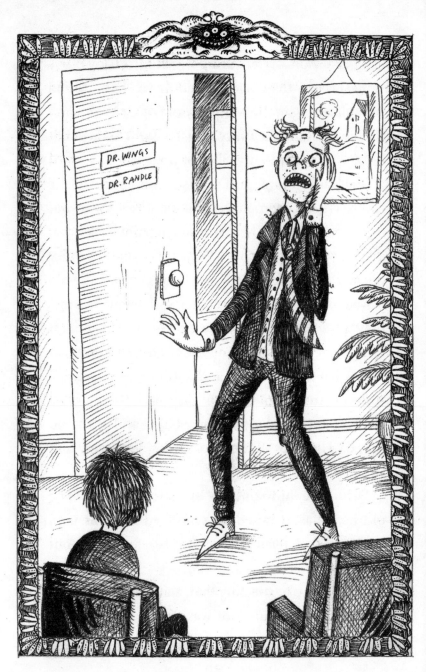

*Dirk smiled at him*

he shifted position so he could listen.

'Extraordinary case,' Dr Wings was saying. 'He still insists some kind of disembodied arm – a child's arm at that – came into his room and shaved his beard off! Astonishing tale! I've never heard anything like it.'

'I know, I know,' said Professor Randle. 'And now he shaves obsessively three times a day, just to make sure there is nothing there for anyone else to shave off, the poor fellow.'

'Indeed – looks painful too!' said Wings.

'Whatever it is, it also cost him his job – and he's convinced that Dirk Lloyd kid had something to do with it,' said Randle.

'Impossible, of course, but I can see why he'd think that,' said Wings.

'I know, that one's even more astonishing than Grousammer! He's up next, by the way.'

'What, the Lector kid?' said Wings.

'Yes, Damien,' said Randle.

'Right, call him in, Randle, call him in,' said Wings.

'What? You're not the boss of me, you call him in!' quipped Randle.

'Oh, I'm not the boss, eh? Who is then – wait, let me guess, someone called Randle, I suppose?'

'Don't start, Wings, or by heaven, I'll...' said Randle, his voice rising.

'What, what, you'll what?' said Wings, getting to his feet noisily.

Dirk raised his eyes. By the Dark Gods, what a pair of psycho fools they were! Better put a stop to this, or he'd be here forever, he thought, so he barged into the room, with a breezy, 'Hello, gentlemen, I'm here!'

Dr Wings was on his feet, jaw jutting out, one hand pointing aggressively at Randle, who was behind his desk, flicking rude signs with both hands at Wings. They both froze.

'Ah, Dirk, come in, come in,' said Wings, sitting back down as if nothing had happened.

'Yes, yes, sit down, sit down,' said Randle pointing at the couch in the middle of the room, between their desks.

'Wine gum?' said Wings, offering a bag of sweets to Dirk. Dirk took a black one, and began to chew.

There followed a tedious hour-long interrogation which went along these lines:

Wings: 'Do you still think your mother was a Vampire Queen from another world and your father a Wizard?'

Dirk: 'Yes.'

Randle: 'Do you want to talk about it?'

Dirk: 'No.'

Wings: 'What were you doing in the woods with your friends?'

Dirk: 'Hiding out with the Winged Demon of Sussex that's been in the news, of course!'

Randle: 'What? Come on, you expect us to believe that?'

Dirk: 'No.'

Wings: 'Are you from another world?'

Dirk: 'Maybe.'

Randle: 'What is it like, that world?'

Dirk: 'Some trees have wine gums as fruit!'

Wings: 'Really? That sounds great!'

Dirk: 'Hah, hah!'

Randle: 'No, Wings you idiot, he's making it up.'

Wings: 'What? I knew that! I knew that, of course I knew that, I was trying to humour him, draw him out, and now you've ruined it, Randle!'

93

*Randle: 'Oh, so now it's my fault is it?'*
*Dirk: 'Hah, hah, hah, this is fun!'*

And so it went on. Eventually, they had to let him go. Dirk had to sit in the waiting room, while Miss Cloy went in to talk to Wings and Randle. Naturally, Dirk sneaked over and put his ear to the key hole.

'A most fascinating case,' said Wings.

'Indeed, going to require a lot of work, a lot!' said Randle.

Dirk raised his eyes. Oh, the horror!

'So,' said Wings, 'next session same time next week, Miss Cloy?'

'Unfortunately, I'm not available then, but we've arranged for you to do a home visit, you can do the session in his room.'

'Good, his room is good – familiar place, home ground, maybe he'll open up a bit,' said Randle.

Dirk groaned aloud at the thought. Too loud! Everything went silent inside the office. Dirk quickly backed off from the door – just as Miss Cloy swept it open. She glared at Dirk suspiciously. Dirk gave her the Shrug of Feigned Innocence.

'What?' he said.

# Skinrash

Back home at last, Dirk summoned Dave to his desk. He unravelled the message and the bottle attached to the Crow's leg. Excitedly, he read it.

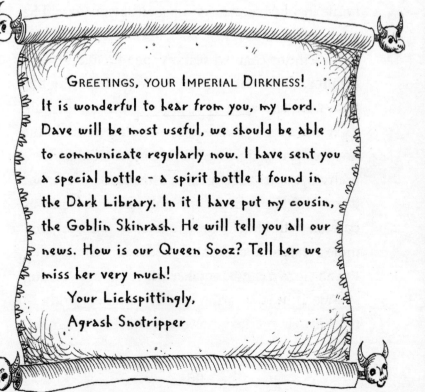

GREETINGS, YOUR IMPERIAL DIRKNESS!

It is wonderful to hear from you, my Lord. Dave will be most useful, we should be able to communicate regularly now. I have sent you a special bottle - a spirit bottle I found in the Dark Library. In it I have put my cousin, the Goblin Skinrash. He will tell you all our news. How is our Queen Sooz? Tell her we miss her very much!

Your Lickspittingly,
Agrash Snotripper

'*Bah*,' said Dirk. 'They seem more concerned about Sooz than me!' Although he had to admit, she had done a good job over there and they did love her for it. Well, a good job if you're into peace and harmony, that is. I mean, who likes that sort of thing? And he was the original Dark Lord, the one and only, as it were, didn't that count for anything?

Anyway, enough of thinking like that. Things to do!

He took the Spirit Bottle (a one-use magical bottle in which creatures – people, even – could be stored inside to reappear later, full size) and carefully flipped the enchanted seal off the top. Out burst a column of thin, wispy green smoke, pouring out like hose water. It began to coalesce in the air, forming itself into a recognisable shape – a little goblin! This one was pretty ugly (to be fair, most Goblins were pretty ugly). Its nose wasn't as long as Agrash's, but it was still fairly prodigious and its green skin was covered with blotchy brown patches, like oversized moles. Hairy moles. Yuk!

The Goblin came together with a gloopy sucking sound. It was wearing a dirty leather jerkin – reassuringly marked, however, with Dirk's symbol, the Great Seal of the Dark Lord – and stained woollen trousers. He had a rusty old Goblin axe, etched with Darklands glyphs, hanging from his belt. He had a leather sack slung over one bony, hairy-moled shoulder. Incongruously, he was wearing a fine pair of blue and white polished leather boots, with bright gold laces.

'Ughh...that was weird,' it said in rough, but slightly squeaky tones. He looked up at Dirk. 'Ah, your Imperial Darkness, greetings from your Iron Tower,' he added.

'Greetings, minion!' said Dirk, 'It is good to see a friendly face around here for once!'

'Thanks, your Throbtasticness,' said the Goblin. 'I'm Agrash's cousin, and me name's Skinrash. Honour to meet yer!'

Skinrash extended a blotchy, hairy, green hand for Dirk to shake. Dirk simply raised an eyebrow.

Skinrash looked puzzled. Dirk nodded at the floor.

'Oh yeah, course! There's me thinkin' you was just an 'ooman kid for a mo!' said Skinrash, as he sank to one knee. 'Skinrash, Goblin minion, at yer service, O my master!'

'That's better!' said Dirk. 'Rise, Skinrash, and report.'

Skinrash got up, wiped his nose, and said, 'Well, your Darkness, Agrash and Skabber are lookin' after fings well enough. With you and the White Wizard – may his hair turn black – bein' away, not much is going on. Everyone's kind of gettin' on wiv stuff, like living and that...'

'Are you suggesting that the Darklands would be better off without us?' said Dirk, slightly annoyed.

'Wot! Nah, never, your Supremeness, never, 'course not! Better off wivout old Whitey, sure, but not you, Master, not you!'

'All right, Skinrash, go on,' said a mollified Dirk, rather enjoying this. It was a bit like old times. After all, Skinrash wasn't to know that Dirk wasn't anything like the old Dark Lord. He was much nicer, for a start. Well, less nasty, certainly.

'Umm... Commonwealth geezers are quiet, a few patrols, but nothing bad. More Orcs come to the tower, Goblinz too. Got a bigger army now. Soozville's still going – some o' them hoomanz moved back in, so they're trading and that. Getting on all right, in fact.'

Dirk folded his arms uncomfortably. Sooz had done well but Dirk couldn't help himself when he thought about her work in the Darklands – it just irritated him. Peace and harmony? *Bah!*

'Enough of that,' said Dirk. 'Have you got any information that is of use to me here, on Earth?'

'Oh yeah,' said Skinrash. 'Agrash gave me stuff to give you!' The goblin reached into his sack and brought out two large white crystals. 'It's a couple of... anafema cysts or somfink,' said the Goblin.

'Aha, two Anathema Crystals! Excellent,' said Dirk, taking them from Skinrash's hands. (The Anathema Crystal, when shattered, propelled nearby people from the Darklands to Earth and turned Dark Lords into human children whilst also sucking out all of their Essence of Evil. That was how Sooz and Chris had 'saved' Dirk the last time – by using a Crystal that had sent the Dark Lord, Chris, Sooz, Gargon and Rufino tumbling through the abyss between the worlds and back down to Earth, where Dirk had changed back into his schoolboy form.)

Dirk held one of them up to the light and examined it closely.

Skinrash said, 'Agrash tol' me to say that these two are the only ones left. He looked up stuff in the Dark Library, but he's not sure if they'll work proper here. Like, will it magic up people all the way back to the

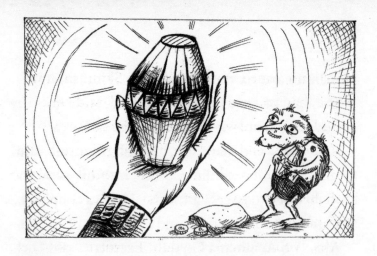

Darklands? Dunno. But still, he reckons it may help.'

'Better here in my hands than sitting in the Iron Tower, that's for sure. Anything else of use?' said Dirk.

'Well, there's these,' said Skinrash, handing Dirk a leather drawstring purse full of gold coins.

'Good! I'm sure I can find a use for them,' said Dirk, pocketing it swiftly. 'Anything else?'

'Well, no, just me, your Coolness. I can be your loyal bodyguard and that, plus I can read and write too, just like me cousin!'

'A nice thought, Skinrash, but the trouble is, I can't really take you round with me, it'd freak out the locals too much. Especially if I took you to school!'

'Skool? What – magic skool? Gladiator skool?' said Skinrash.

'No, no, much worse than that, Skinrash, much worse than you can possibly imagine!' said Dirk.

Suddenly there was a knock on the door.

'Quick, in here!' said Dirk, bundling Skinrash into his clothes cupboard. 'Don't make a sound – and no one, absolutely no one, must lay their eyes on you, ever, got it?'

'Yes, your Hugeness,' said a worried-looking Skinrash, as Dirk shut the cupboard door on him.

'Who is it?' said Dirk. The door opened a little, and Dr Jack Purejoie put his head round the door.

'Dinner's ready, Dirk,' he said.

'Right, I'll be down...' Just then, a loud sneeze sounded from the cupboard, followed by a muffled, 'Eurrgh!'

'What was that?' said Jack, eyebrow raised.

'Xbox game, that's all – I'll be down in a moment,' said Dirk, pushing the door shut, forcing Dr Purejoie to pull his head back rather smartly, with a 'Whoa, steady there!' Dr Jack was kind of used to this sort of behaviour from Dirk by now, so he didn't take it too badly. 'Just don't be too long or it'll get cold,' he added, as he retreated down the stairs.

As soon as he was gone, Dirk yanked the cupboard

door open. 'Cretinous Goblin, I told you to be... Oh no, what have you done!'

Skinrash had sneezed all over Dirk's Grim Reaper dressing gown...covering it in lumpy green snot and stinky Goblin spit.

'Sorry, your Dark Majesty, sorry,' said a shame-faced Skinrash.

~~November 22nd, 2013~~ Rip-out-their-hearts 22nd
*I shall use a crystal as soon as I can. Perhaps we can all go back to the Darklands, where I can leave Rufino and Gargon, and use the second crystal to return to Earth and deal with Hasdruban. Then again, why not stay in the Darklands? Hmm, Sooz might consider it, but would Chris? But I can hardly leave Skinrash on Earth, can I? Skinrash... What am I going to do with a Goblin? Keep him in the cupboard? What do I feed him? And where...arg, I can't even begin to imagine this...where is he going to go to the toilet? Do I have to sneak him into the bathroom? Or...even worse, put a bucket in the cupboard? Who's going to empty it?*

# The Wendle Herald

## Local News

# Another Sighting of the Winged Demon of Sussex

Local school caretaker Darren Cheal, out walking in Willowdown Wood, claims he saw some kind of creature capering about in the trees. He alleges this demonic beast was holding something like a musical instrument. Shortly after the sighting, a terrible noise sprang up. 'Like some kind of thrash metal band literally thrashing metal on metal, accompanied by someone banging on a car roof with a sledgehammer.' Respected psychologists Dr Wings and Mr Randle had this to say on the matter. 'Sound as well as visions? Now that is unusual,' said Dr Wings. 'More like Mr Cheal was on drugs, if you ask me,' said Professor Randle.

Detective Inspector Carwyn Hughes said, 'Bloke in a suit with a guitar, probably.'

~~November 22nd, 2013~~ Rip-out-their-hearts 22nd

*Hah, hah, the blundering fools! I told them this band business wouldn't work. At this rate, they'll be discovered in no time at all. And then what? They'll put Gargon in a lab to experiment on, and Rufino into an asylum for nutters who think they're Paladins from another dimension.*

# *Ambush!*

Dirk struggled on through the streets of Whiteshields, pulling an old cello case behind him that he'd found at the back of the Purejoies' garage and strapped to a wheeled luggage rack. He was huffing and puffing along as the cello case was much heavier than it should have been.

'Are we there yet, your Enormity?' squeaked a muffled voice from inside the cello case.

'No, be silent, Goblin of little wit!' hissed Dirk, glancing over worriedly at the young couple walking by on the other side of the road. Fortunately, they were too wrapped up in each other to notice the talking cello case.

Dirk was transporting Skinrash to the Forest of Demons, where Gargon, Rufino, Sooz and Chris were hanging out doing stupid band stuff. He hoped to use one of the Anathema Crystals to take them all back to the Darklands. Well, Gargon, Rufino, and Skinrash, at any rate – he'd have to discuss who else with Sooz and Chris. He'd considered using a Crystal on the headmaster and the Witch if he could but he wasn't really sure if it was worth it. Hasdruban had probably used some other method of travelling between the planes, so it was possible he'd just come back again by other means, assuming the crystal even worked in the first place. Dirk really needed to deal with Hasdruban, but at this stage there wasn't much he could do, so for now, he would see if he could get Gargon, Rufino and Skinrash away from Earth before they were discovered.

He came to the bridge that led out of town and headed out on a country path. He had to cross a couple of fields to reach the wood. Up ahead, he could see someone out for a walk coming towards him – a tall, thin fellow with a dog. They nodded a greeting as they came together – still, the walker gave him an odd look. What was a kid doing dragging a cello along a country footpath? His dog dashed up to the case and begin sniffing madly.

'Open air school concert in the woods,' said Dirk breezily.

'Uh huh.' The walker nodded.

The dog began barking at the cello case, even trying to bite it, growling and worrying at it.

'Boo! Get back here!' said the walker, yanking the dog onward by its lead. The dog looked up at its master plaintively, as if to say, 'But there's a Goblin in there, I tell you, a Goblin!!!!' As they walked away, the dog looked back and whined.

Dirk hurried on quickly, glancing back nervously, shaking his head. School concert? In November? And why was he dragging it by hand – didn't make sense. And dogs were trouble! Still, the walker didn't seem bothered, so he hurried on.

Finally Dirk reached the edge of the forest. 'Not long, now,' he said to Skinrash.

'Toptastic, for it's gettin' stinky hot in here, your Mightiness!' said Skinrash.

I bet it is, thought Dirk to himself. Last night, Skinrash had unleashed the most hideous fart ever. It'd made Dirk think about putting together some kind of Goblin Gas unit. Feed 'em up with the right stuff – curry and beans? – and they'd be deadly! He'd had to sneak Skinrash to the toilet, but he couldn't really do it safely until the early hours, so he'd had to endure a salvo of stinking horror. If Skinrash had farted inside that cello case – well, being gassed to death by his own noxious emissions was a distinct possibility.

Dirk looked around – he was deep enough in the forest not to be seen from the road, but sometimes people took walks through the woods. There was no one around. It looked like he could let Skinrash out so he could walk the rest of the way. He was leaning over to open the case, when he caught a flash of brightest white against the autumnal yellows and reds of the forest.

Suddenly, out of the foliage, leaped Dr Hasdruban – wearing his usual white suit and hat, white cane in hand. From behind a tree, the White Witch also stepped.

'Dumpsy Deary!' said Dirk. That was the name that Dirk used to call the White Witch when she'd been his nanny, way back when. A nanny sent by Hasdruban to kill him, mind you, but still. Things had changed a lot since then, though, obviously.

'Now we've got you, Evil One!' yelled Hasdruban.

Dirk looked up in surprise, but rapidly regained his composure. 'Oh yeah, and what spell are you going to try now, you old fool?' he said dismissively.

'Spell? I'm not going to bother with magic,' said Dr Hasdruban silkily. He grabbed the top of his cane with his other hand, twisted it until it clicked and drew out a long, thin, steel blade. 'Oh no, this time I'm going to get you once and for all, spawn of evil!'

Dirk's jaw dropped in horror. Two adults, one with a sword, versus a thirteen-year-old boy? No fair. But then again...maybe Dirk could even the odds a little. Quickly he reached for the cello case.

'What, you're going play the cello, and hope to soothe my vengeful rage, is that it, Dark One?' laughed Hasdruban.

'Oh no, better than that,' said Dirk, and he ripped the case open. Out leaped Skinrash with a blast of stinking air. Dirk reeled back in disgust – Hasdruban gagged, staggering for a moment, overcome by the fumes. The White Witch, standing behind him was far enough away not to be affected, though her face, Dirk noted, was a mask of uncertainty. Perhaps she wasn't so keen on the idea of spitting a thirteen-year-old schoolboy with a sword.

'Defend me, my minion, from that murdering

madman, Hasdruban the White!' said Dirk as loud as he could, in the hope Gargon or Rufino were in earshot.

Dr Hasdruban, recovered from the stench-blast, narrowed his eyes. 'A nasty little Goblin!' he said, turning to the White Witch. 'Don't tell me he's just a boy, do boys have Goblin bodyguards, eh? Do they?'

The White Witch gave a noncommittal shrug. Skinrash, meanwhile, blinking in the bright sunlight, took one look at Hasdruban, said, 'Oh no, it's the White Wiz hi-self!' and took to his heels as fast as he could.

Just like that. He was gone.

Dirk couldn't believe it! 'Why, you little...' was all he managed to get out before Hasdruban laughed out loud.

'There is no loyalty amongst the evil,' he said, brandishing his blade.

Dirk thought about turning tail and running too, but instead, thinking fast, he reached into a pocket and drew out one of the Anathema Crystals. Hasdruban leaped forward, Dirk leaped back, and threw the crystal at the Wizard's feet where it shattered, giving off a cloud of wispy, white, diamond-dust smoke.

Hasdruban stopped, surprised.

'What the...? Oh, I see. Hah, clever, Evil One, clever – but not clever enough, I'm afraid! They won't work here on earth, oh no!' With that, he cut at Dirk with the blade. Reflexively, Dirk put an arm up, and the sword sliced down across it.

'Argh!' screamed Dirk.

Hasdruban laughed in triumph, but the White Witch put a hand over her mouth, clearly shocked at the way things were going. Dirk didn't really have time to think about that. He staggered back, bleeding from his arm, as Hasdruban stepped forward again, blade raised high. Dirk, thinking on his feet, whipped his arm forward, unleashing a spray of blood right into Hasdruban's eyes!

'Aiieee!' cried the Wizard, temporarily blinded. That gave Dirk a moment's respite. He was about to run, when suddenly a huge figure crashed down out of the sky to land between Hasdruban and Dirk.

'Gargon, thank the Dark Gods!' sighed Dirk.

'You no kill my master!' bellowed Gargon with a voice like iron filings in a blender turned up to eleven. Hasdruban, desperately trying to clear his

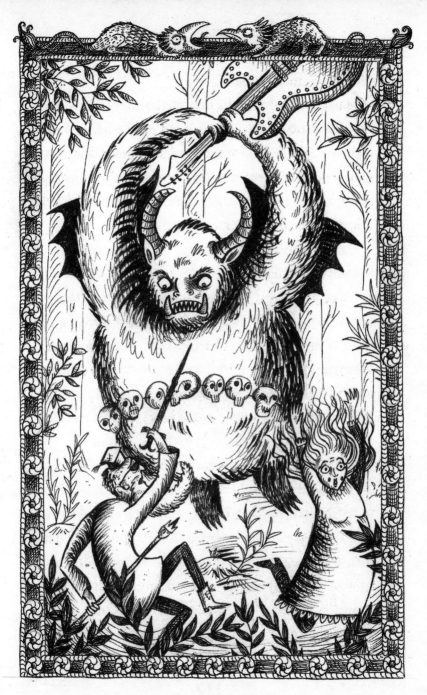

*Death by guitar*

vision, squinted up at Gargon.

'Get ye gone, foul demon of the night!' he cried, raising one hand and gesturing as if casting some kind of spell. The White Witch darted forward, angry now, ready to defend her master. Rufino also came running onto the scene, followed by Chris and Sooz close behind.

'Hah, your White Words, your so-called holy magic won't work here, Hasdruban! Gargon will tear you to pieces!' shouted a triumphant Dirk.

Gargon roared again, and raised his weapon high over his head to bring it crashing down on Hasdruban's skull. Dirk looked up at Gargon with gleeful relish and anticipation. Now that meddling Wizard would pay for cutting him! No one cuts the Dark Lord and gets away with it!

But then Dirk saw what Gargon had in his hands. A large guitar...

'Wait, Gargon, NO!' said Dirk, coming to his senses. Everyone froze for a moment. The headmaster, face splattered with blood, looking more like an old man than a great Wizard, thin cane sword held up in pitiful defence, the White Witch, moving in front of him, trying to shield him, a huge winged demon, face a mask of murderous intent, raised arms ready to crush the old man, and Rufino rushing in, with two children behind him.

'No, we can't do this, Gargon,' continued Dirk.

Gargon frowned. 'What you mean? It's him, Hasdruban. We never get this chance again, Gargon smash him!'

'No, no, he's also the headmaster. We can't... I mean, I'm not the Dark...it's Earth...you know,' said Dirk tailing off in confusion.

Hasdruban stared at Dirk in amazement. The White Witch began scribbling a note.

Sooz said, 'He's right, Gargon. We can't beat the headmaster to death with a guitar. It's just not done.'

'If my Queen say so, then Gargon agree,' he said, and he lowered the guitar.

The White Witch handed a note to Hasdruban, who barely noticed. He was staring at Dirk in astonishment, as if he couldn't believe what he'd just heard.

'What? Oh!' he said, taking the note. Quickly he read it. He frowned for a moment, but then he turned to the White Witch and spat out, 'Hah, how can he be just a boy? Look, he's got Gargon with him. Gargon!'

Meanwhile, Rufino, Sooz and Chris rushed over to Dirk, who was swaying on his feet. Quickly, Rufino began bandaging up Dirk's arm.

'It's not deep, just a flesh wound,' said Rufino, 'no need to worry. Well, unless...' and he flicked a glance over at Hasdruban. 'Was the cane sword poisoned?' he asked.

Hasdruban looked over at him, a look of contempt on his face. '*Bah*, the traitor speaks. No, of course not. I am the White Wizard, I do not use poison!'

'That's not what I heard,' said Dirk loudly. 'I mean, what happened to the last White Wizard, the one you took over from? What did he die of?'

'How dare you! I'll kill you, kill you!!!' shrieked Hasdruban, stepping forward, but Gargon blocked his way and growled.

'Bit sensitive about that, are we?' said Dirk with a grin, despite the pain he was suffering.

Hasdruban gritted his teeth angrily. But then he looked up at Gargon, blinked, and stepped back.

'Mexican standoff,' said Chris.

'Yeah,' said Sooz. 'Nothing else is going to

happen here – I say we all walk away. We take our wounded boy, you go home.'

Hasdruban took a white hanky from his pocket and began to clean the blood of his face. The White Witch tugged at his sleeve, nodding.

Hasdruban shook his head, uncertain.

'I could have you killed, you know. Here and now,' said Dirk.

'Think about that,' said Sooz, worried that Dirk might change his mind and decide to do just that. 'Think about it, and maybe we can come to a truce, or peace even. Peace would be good, don't you think?'

The White Witch nodded even more vigorously. Hasdruban looked at her, frowning angrily. He put a hand up to his head, thinking.

But then slashed it down emphatically. '*Bah*, Witch, you have become weak,' he shouted into her face, before turning to Dirk and the rest. 'As for you, this is some kind of trick. You're scared! Scared of what would happen if you murdered the headmaster and his deputy, scared of the humans and their "policemen", that is all!'

'No,' said Sooz, 'he's changed, he really has, he's

not the Dark Lord any more!'

'Oh, please, why should I listen to you? The Moon Queen? Wielder of the Great Ring? You are as corrupt as he, both of you, children of darkness, you are, steeped in evil! No, better to destroy you utterly, for the benefit of all!'

Dirk shook his head in despair. 'It's useless, Sooz,' he said. 'He's quite mad!'

The White Witch pulled on Hasdruban's sleeve, trying to drag him away. Hasdruban, glancing over at Gargon and Rufino, allowed himself to be led but not before he'd got one final word in.

'This isn't finished, oh no,' he shouted, 'not finished at all!'

# A Gobbling Goblin

At last Dirk made it back to his room, the earthly equivalent of his Inner Sanctum in the Iron Tower. He leaned back against the door and rubbed his arm. It was painful but he'd had worse. Twelve stitches. All done by Dr Jack at home. Dirk had claimed he'd been cutting some bread and slipped, slicing his arm on the bread knife. But he'd overheard Mr and Mrs Purejoie talking about him afterwards, and worrying that maybe he'd done it himself to get attention or something. Hah! Dark Lords don't harm themselves, it's other people they harm, didn't they realise that? Still, no doubt they'd

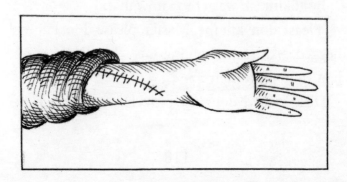

tell Wings and Randle about it, and they'd start asking stupid questions about why and when he'd started and all the rest.

A sudden noise from the cupboard caught Dirk's attention. A kind of snuffling, gobbling sound. Skinrash! 'That little...' muttered Dirk as he wrenched the door open. And there was the Goblin, blinking up at him, mouth stuffed with chocolate cake.

Dirk narrowed his eyes. 'You coward!' he said accusingly.

Skinrash cringed down into the corner of the cupboard. 'I know, I know, I'm sorry, your Majesticness, but I'm only a poor little gobber and old Whitey – he can blast twenny gobbers into pieces wiv his staff! I seen it!'

Dirk sighed. That was true. He'd seen it as well. Except that his terrible magic didn't work here on earth.

But Skinrash wasn't to know that.

'Please don' kill me, Master, please don' kill me!' begged Skinrash, holding his chocolate-covered hands up pleadingly.

Dirk looked down at him. His warty face was

covered in chocolate – it was even stuck to the hair on his moles. And his knees were shaking. The poor little fellow was greedy, yes, but also obviously terrified. Dirk shook his head. Once, when he had been an actual Dark Lord he might well have killed him. Or put him in the Dungeons of Doom or something. But now, he just didn't have the heart.

'Oh, stop it, Skinrash, really. I won't kill you, I promise.'

Skinrash darted forward and hugged Dirk around the knees. 'Thank you, Master, thank you for sparing poor old Skinrash!' he burbled.

Dirk closed his eyes in resigned dismay. His trousers were now thoroughly smeared with chocolate.

'Where did you get the cake from?' said Dirk.

'Downstairs cupboard,' said Skinrash.

'Did anyone see you?' said Dirk, unable to suppress a grin. Goblins were just naughty chaos bringers, really. And Dark Lords quite liked chaos.

'More importantly,' added Dirk, 'did anyone see you in the town? How'd you get back here?'

'Over the 'oomans' rooftops, your Ultimateness,' said Skinrash with rising confidence, now that he

119

was sure he wasn't going to be punished. 'No one saw me, no one at all, I made sure of it, Dark Master!'

'OK, then Skinrash. I forgive you, though it'll be me that gets the blame for stealing the cake, I'll bet,' said Dirk.

'Maybe you can blame that other kid,' said Skinrash. 'That's the Darklands way, after all, your Supreme Evilness.'

'Hah, hah, yes it is, Skinrash. Good idea! Now get back in that cupboard. It's time for bed, and I'm exhausted.'

'Bad day, eh, Sire?'

'I'll say! I've dragged a Goblin in a cello case halfway across town, had my arm hacked open by a crazed Wizard from another world and then stitched up again by my foster-father who thinks I did it to myself deliberately, and after all that, I get smeared with sticky chocolate. I think that counts as a bad day, don't you?'

~~November 23rd, 2013~~ Rip-out-their-hearts 23rd
*Issue two of the* Dark Times *available now!*

# *THE DARK TIMES*

Issue Two          Price: 5 Copper Christophers

*'My name is Dirk but you may call me Master.'*
Dirk Lloyd

## *Today's Horrorscope*

~~*Virgo Good-for-sacrifices*~~ – Today, I predict that
you will read your horoscope. Amazingly, it
will tell you what you are doing at this precise
moment! You are reading your horoscope.
~~*Sagittarius*~~ *Arrow-in-the-heart* – Whatever
you do, don't eat a banana today! If you do,
it will explode, leaving your mouth and face
covered in unpleasant banana mush, and then
people will laugh at you. If they aren't already,
of course.
~~*Pisces*~~ *Stinkyfish* – You are slowly turning into
a fish. Soon, you will feel an uncontrollable
urge to swim in the sea. You will do so and

never be seen again by humankind. Examine your neck. How are those gills coming along?

*Aquarius Waterygrave* – Be careful, for there is a wormhole in space-time near where you are walking. If you step on it, you will be propelled to an alien planet where giant molluscs with helium filled shells float in a steamy sky and the earth is covered in a carpet of squidworms. You will not like it. Not only that, you'll miss dinner.

*Capricorn Smellygoat* – You will get a job. Maybe not today, but someday. Probably. Who says horoscopes aren't accurate?

## *Letters with the Aunt of Agony*

Dear Aunt of Agony,
My dad appears to be mutating into some kind of half man, half frog creature. I am worried now that it might happen to me. What shall I do?
Yours,
Kermit Webfoot

*Dear Kermit,*
*Don't worry, I know all about your family, the*
*Webfoots. It's quite normal for you guys to turn*
*into frogs, as you're all a bunch of mutant freaks.*
*Just try not to eat too many flies, they're really*
*unsanitary.*
*Yours Sneeringly,*
*The Aunt of Agony*

Dear Aunt of Agony,
I have recently taken over the headmastership
of a large comprehensive. However, some of the
pupils are so difficult to deal with, that I can't
seem to clear my head to think. What should I do?
Yours,
Dr Hasdruban

*Dear Dr Hasdruban*
*Stick your head down the toilet and flush it. That*
*will clear your mind. Trust me, it works.*
*Yours Sneeringly,*
*The Aunt of Agony*

Dear Aunt of Agony,
How do I make a potion of mind control?
Yours,
Laura Wibblebottom

*Dear Laura*
*A handful of Hogweed, harvested at midnight on All Soul's Eve, some ground-up bonemeal of a convict hanged at a crossroads (any part of the skeleton will do), a little salt water, and three feathers from a Storm Crow.*
*Yours Sneeringly,*
*The Aunt of Agony*
*ps Good luck with finding that lot!*

This issue of the *Dark Times* brought to you by the Great Dirk!

Yours Unfaithfully,

*I, the Dark Lord, Master of the Legions of Dread and Sorcerer Supreme, etc etc*

# This Time, Chris Gets Stitched Up

The next morning, Dirk made his way downstairs for breakfast, nursing his bandaged arm. Dirk paused by the dining room. Mr and Mrs Purejoie were in deep conversation with Chris.

'We know it was you,' said Mrs Purejoie.

'No, no, it wasn't,' said Chris emphatically.

'It's really hurtful that you'd lie to us like this, Christopher!' said Dr Purejoie. 'After all, we found the remains of the cake in your room.'

'You could have just asked us for cake, you didn't have to steal it, dear,' said Mrs Purejoie. 'But what's worse is lying about it.'

Dirk walked on by, trying not to attract any attention. Chris spotted him, though, and stared at him, eyes narrowing. Dirk couldn't help himself and the corner of his mouth went up. It was all he could do to stop himself from laughing out loud.

'Well, what have you got to say for yourself?' said Dr Purejoie.

Chris sighed. Dirk had obviously tricked him. Better to just get it over with. He said, 'All right, it was me! I did it, I took the cake, stuffed it all, and left a bit in my drawer. Of course I did. Now, can I go please?'

'All right, then, Chris, at least you came clean about it,' said Mrs Purejoie, 'But we're not done yet. It is time for school, and we have to go to work, but we're going to have to talk about this later.'

The Purejoies, faces solemn and serious, as if Chris had been arrested for robbing a bank or something, got the children ready for school. The whole time, Chris stared at Dirk suspiciously, whilst it took all of Dirk's Dark Lord willpower not to laugh and laugh and laugh.

'So,' said Chris, once they were on their own and walking to school. 'Thanks for stitching me up – very funny. But why? That's what I don't get.'

'I'm sorry, Chris, but I had to deflect attention from me – and Skinrash,' said Dirk.

'Skin rash? What rash? A curse-from-Hasdruban type rash?'

And Dirk explained to Chris about Skinrash the Goblin, how he'd used the Essence to create his Shadowshades, how Agrash had sent him a Spirit Bottle, and that he'd got a Goblin hiding in the cupboard and how Skinrash had run off and then stolen the cake and stuffed it all just like a typical Goblin.

'You could have told me about it first,' said Chris. 'I'd probably have taken the rap rather than have Mum and Dad finding a Goblin in your cupboard, I get that that would be bad, I'm not stupid, you know!'

'More fun, this way,' said Dirk.

'Right, I see,' said Chris. 'I'm just a worthless lackey, I get it.'

'No, no, I didn't mean it like that. Anyway, I never got the chance to tell you what with everything going on,' said Dirk.

But Chris didn't reply. In fact, he never said a word for the rest of the journey to school, despite Dirk's attempts to start a conversation.

# A Black Hag?

Dirk's arm was healing up nicely. Hasdruban hadn't made his presence known for a few days now – no doubt he was planning something new, although in the meantime he had arranged for Dirk to be hit with a lot of extra homework. Sooz claimed her band was coming along well. She'd called them Soozie and the Nightwalkers. Gargon on lead guitar, Rufino on drums, Chris on bass, and Sooz as lead singer. She'd asked Dirk to come and listen to them rehearse in the woods, but he wasn't that interested. Anyway, he didn't have much time what with detentions and the homework and the rest.

It was late afternoon and Dirk was walking down a deserted school corridor near the music room, a shed load of extra homework under one arm, getting ready to go home. Suddenly, he saw something that made him pull up short. Before him stood a figure dressed in black rags, with a ripped-up black lace veil over her face, and a kind of Gothic bridal headdress of black rags covered in wispy cobwebs on her head. Her feet were bare, but covered in black dirt. Long black tattered gloves covered her arms, and her hands ended in long black nails, like iron talons.

'By the Dark Gods, 'tis the Lady Grieve!' said Dirk to himself in amazed tones. What was she doing here?

The Lady Grieve, or the Black Hag, as she was known, was an ancient witch-assassin who lived in the Darklands, the counterpart of the White Witch of Holy Vengeance – they were the deadliest of enemies, implacably opposed to each other, a vendetta that had lasted for hundreds of years. The Black Hag could be hired to kill people using her long, black nails, for they were covered in a horrible poison. Dirk, when he'd been the Dark Lord, had actually used her once or twice, but it was a long time ago. Summoning her was complicated and her payment was difficult to get.

Dirk walked up to her excitedly. She was quite

thoroughly evil and a true servant of the dark –
maybe she'd be an ally or something, or perhaps
she had been sent by Agrash to help him!

'Greetings, Lady Grieve, it is I, the Dark Lord!'
said Dirk, forgetting that he was, of course, just a
human boy.

The Lady Grieve turned to look at him. She
appeared surprised. Before she could say anything,
Sooz marched out of the music room. She was
wearing her full Moon Queen outfit, a black veil of
her own, a long black dress with a silver threaded
bodice, and a beautiful silvery tiara on her head –
all finished off with big, chunky Goth boots.

'Hi, Roanna,' said Sooz, 'great fancy dress outfit!
What are you?'

'Kind of a Goth witch, I guess, though Dirk called
me...what was it you said, Dirk?' said Roanna, for
that is who she really was. Roanna Lynsey. A Goth
friend of Sooz's in fancy dress, and not the Black
Hag at all. Of course!

'Umm...nothing, my mistake,' said Dirk,
embarrassed.

'But it was cool – the Lady Grief or something,'
said Roanna.

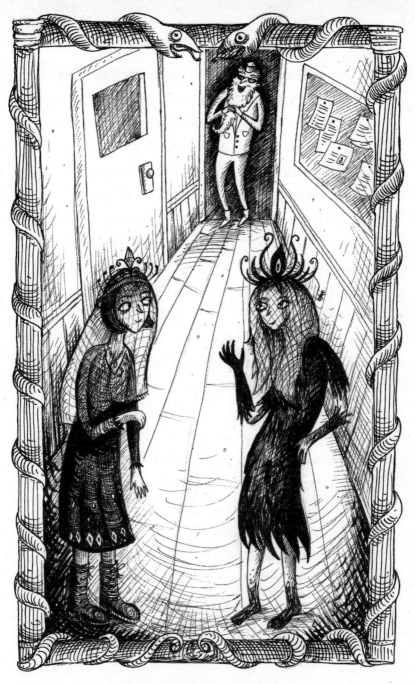

*Sooz and Roanna, chillin'*

'Heh, sounds good,' said Sooz. 'So, you're ready for the Goth ball after school?'

'Oh yes,' Roanna replied. 'Your band is playing, isn't it?'

'Yeah,' said Sooz, 'I can't wait, you're going to be blown away by our lead guitarist! You're coming, right, Dirk?'

But Dirk wasn't paying attention. He was staring at the other end of the corridor. For standing there was Hasdruban himself. Dirk frowned. Hasdruban wasn't looking at Dirk, his attention was fixed on Roanna Lynsey. Suddenly, Hasdruban grabbed his beard with both hands, shouted, 'Eureka!' and dashed away out of sight.

'Dirk? Gargon will be there. Playing in public, pretending to be dressed in...' Sooz paused, flicking a glance at Roanna. 'I mean dressed in a monster suit. You know, for the first time,' said Sooz. She tugged at his sleeve, trying to get Dirk's attention but he was lost in a world of his own.

Dirk stared down at the floor, thinking furiously. Hasdruban had recognised the Lady Grieve just as he had. Could he be thinking about hiring the real Black Hag? Surely not! The White Wizard, using the Black Hag? But then again, he would stop at nothing to destroy the Dark Lord, even if it meant consorting with evil – you know, fighting fire with fire and all that. If that was the case, maybe Dirk should get in first, hire her to bump off Hasdruban!

'Oh forget it then – come on Roanna,' said Sooz, shaking her head, and they both went on their way, leaving Dirk to his thoughts.

Dirk was desperately trying to remember what he could about the Black Hag. She lived in a warren of caves, where she kept pictures of all her victims on the walls. From time to time, she would take a picture down, and cry over it, shedding black tears, grieving in some kind of twisted, sick parody of sorrow for her victims. That's why they called her the Lady Grieve. She killed to grieve.

Creepy!

What was it you needed to hire the Black Hag? A picture of the victim drawn in their blood, a special gem of some kind. And something else, something to do with the unicorn. It was tricky for Dark Lords, that one, because to get a unicorn you need a maiden of pure heart. Not many maidens in the Darklands were pure of heart, that was for sure, and there weren't any unicorns. Sooz was pure of heart, though, she could do it, assuming they could find a unicorn. Dirk looked up, but Sooz was long gone.

Suddenly, Dirk realised something and a chill ran down his spine. A picture painted with the blood of the victim? Hasdruban had plenty of his blood from that episode in the woods, he was halfway there already! And he could get a unicorn – plenty of those in Arboretum, the City of the Elves in the Commonwealth of Good Folk, not to mention plenty of pure-hearted, do-gooding Elf maidens.

Is this what he could expect next, an attack from the Black Hag? He'd better be on his guard then, for her talons were coated with a deadly poison. One scratch was usually fatal. Dirk had to get home, send a message to Agrash telling him to search the Dark Library for everything he could find about the Black Hag. He hurried home as fast as he could. The Black Hag was dangerous indeed.

Back in his room, he tossed his homework on the desk, and summoned Dave the Storm Crow. As he did so, a long nose poked out of the cupboard and sniffed the air.

'Is dat you, your Fantasticness?' said Skinrash.

'What? Oh yes, yes, it's safe to come out, Skinrash,' said Dirk, busily writing up a message to send to Agrash.

'I'm starving, Master,' said Skinrash. 'Got sumfink to eat?'

Dirk paused and raised his eyes. He'd forgotten to get food for Skinrash. Having a Goblin in your cupboard was a real pain!

'Hold on, Skinrash,' said Dirk.

Dirk finished his message, tied it to the Crow's leg, and then put on his Shadowshades. The window to the Darklands opened before him, and off went Dave, cawing loudly.

Dirk took off his Shadowshades, and put them away. He looked over at the Goblin and sighed. He had masses of homework to do, but Skinrash really did need to be fed, so he set off for the corner shop.

He returned some time later with dinner for Skinrash. Dirk knew a lot about Goblins, and he'd picked just the right kind of food. Skinrash tucked in noisily and appreciatively.

'Fanx, your Gloryness, this is fantastic!' he said between mouthfuls. Dirk looked down in mild disgust at his plate of tinned corned beef all mashed up with cat biscuits, brussel sprouts and custard.

'Num, nummity num!' mumbled the Goblin. Dirk shook his head and reached for his homework. A splat on the wall startled him. Skinrash had hurled a custard covered sprout, and it had stuck to the wall, slowly dribbling down it.

'Hur, hur, hur,' chortled the Goblin. To be fair, throwing your food around was a sign of appreciation in Goblin culture, but still.

'Stop that!' hissed Dirk.

'But this nosh in a can wiv yellow pus stuff is delish, your Uberness!' said Skinrash.

'Throwing your food around here will only get us both in trouble, so don't do it!' said Dirk.

'Yes, your Strictness,' muttered a crestfallen Skinrash. 'When we goin' home, my Lord? I hate it 'ere in 'oomanland! Not worth even these flash boots wot Agrash gave me.'

Just then, Dirk's DarkPhone rang. He looked at it in surprise. Hardly anyone had that number! He picked it up. Blood red letters appeared on its shadowy surface. 'Sooz, Dark Mistress of the Tower and Queen of the Darklands'. Dirk frowned in irritation at that – he was the rightful ruler of the

Darklands, not her!

He picked up the phone and put it to his ear. Little bony hands reached out from the phone and grabbed his ear, clasping it to the phone. A long arm extended itself from the other side and grabbed his other ear, perfectly placing the phone in front of his mouth. Dirk put his hands down – it was hands-free, of course. He'd designed it that way.

'Hi, Sooz,' he said.

'Hi, Dirk,' said Sooz. 'How's your arm?'

'Fine, aches a bit, but basically fine. I've had worse.'

There was a pause, each unsure what to say next – things hadn't been quite right between them ever since Dirk had used her as a human shield.

'Well,' said Dirk, 'What do you want? I've got a mountain of homework that madman Hasdruban gave me.'

'What do I want? I want you to come to the school concert, that's what I want! Like you said you would,' said Sooz.

'Oh yeah,' said Dirk, 'I'd forgotten about that.'

'How could you forget? Really, Dirk, what's the matter with you? Gargon is playing. In front of loads of people, not to mention Rufino, you need to be there!' said Sooz.

Dirk tsked in irritation. 'The headmaster tried to hack me to pieces with a sword, and now I'm pretty sure that he's going to send one of the deadliest assassins known to Orc, Elf, Man or Beast after me! That's what's wrong with me, little Miss Rock moon!'

Sooz couldn't help herself and giggled. 'Rock moon?'

'Errr. Rock...star, I mean. Rockstar,' said Dirk. 'You know...'

'Yeah, I know. Anyway, maybe you're right. Who is this assassin dude, anyway?'

'The Black Hag. She's got...well, I'll tell you about it later, I've sent a message to Agrash to find out everything he can about her in the Dark Library.'

'OK, and I'll do everything I can to help. But she's not coming tonight, right?' said Sooz.

'No, no, it'll take a few days for Hasdruban to sort things out, I would think, at least,' said Dirk.

'Well, then, please, please come. I so want you to see us play – we're not bad – in fact, Gargon is actually quite good, and I wrote the songs

138

and everything!'

'But I hate all that human music stuff, and I've got so much homework to do!' said Dirk.

Sooz paused for a moment, thinking. Then she said, 'Don't you think you'd better be there, in case something goes wrong? I mean, we'll need your superior brain, and your leadership skills and that.'

'Oh very clever, Sooz, very clever with the flattery! But I suppose you may be right,' said Dirk, looking over at Skinrash who was spilling cat biscuits and custard all over the floor.

'Brill! Get down here as fast as you can, dude, we're up in half an hour!' With that she rang off.

Dirk put the phone down. 'Skinrash, you can read and write, yes?'

'Oh yes, your Blackheartedness, I can! Not as brainy as me cousin Agrash, but still, pretty much a genius for a Goblin!' said Skinrash.

'Right then. I have to go – whilst I'm gone, you can do this homework here,' said Dirk, pointing at the small pile of papers on his desk.

Skinrash blinked up at him. 'Homework? I can do that, your Evilness, no problem!'

*Incredibly, Soozie and the Nightwalkers were a great success! Admittedly, it sounded like a bunch of Orcish blacksmiths, accompanied by a trio of braying demon-donkeys to me, but the humans seemed to like it. Most of them were in 'Goth' fancy dress, which made me nostalgic for home, actually, so that was nice. And they really believed Gargon was a guy in a suit, just like that band Morti! Chris wore his leather Darklands gear, and Sooz looked great in full Goth regalia! One song Sooz wrote was a boy meets girl thing, except the girl was like a Vampire and the boy was a Dark Lord. I liked it! Well, those words I could actually hear at any rate.*

# The School Concert

## An Interview with Soozie and the Nightwalkers

By Lucy Futtock-Brown of *New Rock Magazine* (Lucy was head girl back in 2003).

Whiteshields school held its 15th annual open mike school concert, where pupils can get up on stage and do their stuff. The theme this year was 'Goth'. The highlight of the show was Susan Black's band, Soozie and the Nightwalkers. Afterwards, I spoke to the band.

*Lucy*: Hi, guys, great performance, and great outfits! What musical style would you call yourselves?

*Sooz*: Thanks, Lucy! We call it 'Demonic Goth.'

*Lucy*: Those outfits look so real! I mean, the guitarist...what's his name?

*Guitarist*: Me called Gargon!

*Lucy*: Oh my, what a voice you have!

*Christopher Purejoie*: It's a...a modulator. A special thing in the suit, you know, makes his voice like that.

*Lucy*: Wow! And the teeth! They look so real... I mean...the fangs... and the—

*Gargon*: RWAOORRR!

*Lucy*: Arrrgghhhh!

# Dark Thoughts

Dirk had just handed his homework in (well, Skinrash's homework) and now he stood alone in the school corridor. It was break time, and everyone else was in the playground. Dirk, though, was deep in thought re-reading the message he'd got this morning from Agrash about the Black Hag. It seemed you needed a unicorn's horn, a shadow opal, which was a rare gem found only in the Abyssal Gulfs, and the picture of the target painted in his blood as the price for the Black Hag's services. There was no way Dirk could get any of those here on Earth. It would be hard enough even if he was in the Darklands. But Hasdruban could. He already had some of Dirk's blood – and the chances were that he had the rest just sitting in one of his storerooms in the White Tower. For all he knew, Hasdruban and the White Witch could travel back and forth from Earth to the Commonwealth of Good Folk virtually at will.

Dirk had to assume the worst. He should expect a sudden poison attack from the Lady Grieve at some time in the next few days. The poison consisted of Black Oleander mixed with Nightshade and Hemlock tainted with some unknown evil, according to Agrash, although he was still researching it. The Lady Grieve herself was immune to it, though some scrolls and tomes in the Library claimed that only one other was immune – or at least somewhat resistant – to her poison and that was her counterpart, the White Witch of Holy Vengeance. Interesting, but not much help if they were working together against you, right?

The Lady Grieve wasn't exactly a dangerous fighter in the traditional sense, but she didn't need to be. She used stealth and surprise and speed – all it took was one scratch, and you'd be paralysed, slowly dying, whilst she knelt over you, and 'grieved' for you. Horrible!

No, what he needed was an antidote. Maybe he could send Dave the Crow to Agrash to get the ingredients in the Darklands, and bring them back to them... He could work on it in the chemistry lab, maybe find a cure. Yes, an antidote was the answer!

Dirk looked up. There was Sooz, waving at him. Thank the Dark Gods they were back on speaking terms – she was in a much better mood after the concert had gone so well, and she seemed to have forgiven him for...well, using her as a shield sort of thing. Dirk grimaced at the thought of it. He waved back. It was time for science class with Batty Barnes.

# Wine Gums and Storm Crows

'Rat-a-tat-tat!' sounded loudly on Dirk's bedroom door. Quickly, he put away his Shadowshades, shooed Skinrash into the cupboard and went over to open it. Luckily, Dave the Storm Crow was away on a mission in the Darklands, so he didn't need to worry about that.

'Ah, the Lector kid,' said Dr Wings as Dirk swung the door open.

'What the unprofessionally indiscreet Dr Wings really means is, of course, greetings to the young Dirk!' said Professor Randle with false hilarity and a waspish glance at his colleague.

Dirk sighed. A Wings and Randle therapy session, what a nightmare!

'Greetings, inferior humans!' said Dirk and he smiled up at them. They both blinked uncertainly.

'Do you think we need another adult in the room?' said Randle.

Dr Wings hesitated for a moment. Then, 'No, no, he's just a kid. We'll be fine. Won't we?'

Randle nodded, 'Yes of course, of course. Now...shall we?' he said, showing his partner into the room.

They had chairs with them that they set up in the middle of the room. Dirk was forced to make himself comfortable, lying back on the bed as if were on a psychiatrists' couch.

'Well, Dirk,' said Randle, 'we've heard a lot about you from the headmaster, Dr Hasdruban, and from your father, Dr Purejoie.'

'Indeed,' said Wings, leaning forward. 'Wine gum?' he said, holding out a bag.

Dirk ignored the offer. 'What has that fanatical old fool been saying about me?' he said.

Wings blinked at him. 'What – your father or the headmaster?'

'Hasdruban, of course!' said Dirk crossly.

Wings narrowed his eyes. Randle smiled broadly.

'Oh, lots, lots indeed,' said Randle.

Wings tried to gloss over things. 'Are you sure

you won't have a wine gum, Dirk? Dr Hasdruban has become very fond of them, you know. Very fond indeed!' he said.

'Yeah, developed quite a liking for them, just like Wings here,' said Randle distastefully.

'Really? Well, there's no accounting for taste,' said Dirk.

'Anyway, we haven't come here to talk about wine gums, now, have we, eh?' said Randle.

'No, no, of course not,' said Wings slipping the bag back into his pocket. 'Dr Hasdruban tells us that you were found in the Science lab making a home-made gun.'

'What?' said Dirk. 'That's completely untrue!' And it was untrue. Sure, Dirk probably could make a gun, but it was ridiculously risky. If he was caught... well, juvenile detention centre? Shipped off to a special school? Not to mention all the unwanted attention. He narrowed his eyes. So that was his game, eh? Spreading rumours and lies about him! Cunning old devil!

'Come, come, Dirk, there's no need to lie to us, we're on your side, my boy,' said Wings.

'Tell us, Damien...I mean, Dirk! Tell us, why the

gun? Are you angry about something? Would you like to tell us about it?' said Randle.

'Yeah, sure I'm angry – the headmaster is really the White Wizard and he's out to kill me. See what he did to my arm? He hacked it open with a sword!' said Dirk, holding out his bandaged arm.

'Now, Dirk, please, you can't really expect us to believe that the headmaster is really a wizard from another world who attacked you with a sword, now can you?' said Wings.

Dirk had no answer to that. He didn't expect them to believe him, no. In fact, all he wanted to do was to get this over with as quickly as possible so he could find out what Dave had brought back for him from Agrash in the Darklands.

'We know that you did that to yourself, Dirk, your father told us,' said Randle.

'Foster father!' said Dirk without thinking.

'Ah, is that it? You're angry about being fostered, maybe want to see your own father?' said Wings.

'And that's why you're self-harming? Now we're getting somewhere!' said Randle.

Dirk raised his eyes – what a pair of simpletons! And then he noticed something. The cupboard door inched open...and out came a long, green nose. It sniffed the air...

Dirk stared in fascination. Wings and Randle followed his gaze – the nose retracted in an instant before they could see anything. Dirk looked back at them. He sighed.

'Yes, yes, that's it, I cut myself because I miss my real parents...' said Dirk. If he just agreed with everything they said, it would be over all the sooner, though he added under his breath, 'Notwithstanding the fact that my real parents have been dead for thousands of years.'

Dirk saw something out of the corner of his eye.... A knobbly green and hairy arm, reaching out from inside the cupboard. His heart began to beat. What if they turned round now...

Dirk felt a terrible urge to giggle.

'What about the gun, Dirk, do you want to talk about that?' said Wings.

'The gun? An obvious cheap lie from that madman Hasdruban...umm...wait... Oh, all right, yes, I was going to...errr...shoot it off! You know, somewhere safe, of course. Just to get attention, and that,' said Dirk, though why anyone in the world would do that just to get attention escaped him. Humans were weird, though, they'd probably believe it.

Skinrash's hand was getting closer and closer to Wings' jacket pocket.

'Aha! I knew it,' said Randle. 'This is excellent work, Dirk, we are really going places now!'

Dirk choked out a laugh, as Skinrash's hand darted into Wings' pocket, plucked out the bag of sweets and disappeared back into the cupboard.

Wings frowned. 'What's so funny, Dirk?' he said, oblivious to the loss of his precious wine gums.

'Oh, nothing, nothing,' said Dirk.

Suddenly, a small black spot appeared out of nowhere in the air between the three of them. Dirk looked up at it in panic. Wings and Randle stared in astonishment. It grew a little bigger, and then, with a loud popping noise, Dave the Storm Crow flew into the room. It circled about, flapping wildly, cawed like a tormented soul, and then flew out the window. The black spot winked out.

Wings and Randle continued to stare open mouthed. Dirk couldn't help himself and giggled a bit.

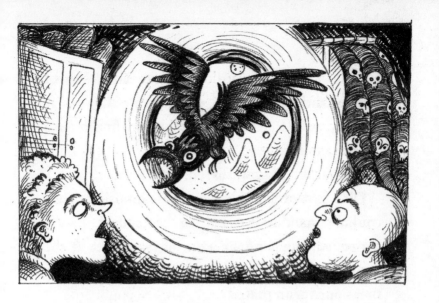

Wings stuttered, 'What in blue...'

'....blazes was that!' finished Randle.

Dirk pulled himself together. He had to bluff this one out. 'Just a bird,' he said. 'A crow – lives on the roof over the road, comes in here from time to time, flies around and out again,' said Dirk, staring at them. How were they going to react?

'Right,' said Wings. 'Yes, of course, just flew in through the window...'

'Yeah,' said Randle. 'Must have. *Must have*. I mean, I didn't see... Umm... Wings, did you see...a...'

Wings stared at him. 'No, can't have. Can't have seen a...thing... No, I saw a crow fly in through the window and out again, that's all.'

'Yes, of course you did. And so did I! Yes, of course,' said Randle.

'Now, well...that's settled...' said a still flummoxed Wings.

'Onwards and upwards, eh?' said Randle.

Dirk smiled a wry smile. Most amusing. They couldn't handle it! Had to pretend it hadn't happened. What a pair. Dirk glanced over at the cupboard. It'd be fun to let Skinrash out, see how they coped with that...

But no, that might be pushing it a bit.

'Anyway, I think our time is done here, don't you, Wings?' said Randle.

'Quite so, quite so,' said Wings, as they got up together to leave. 'We'll see you next time, young man.'

As they moved to the door, Wings reached into his pocket for a wine gum. But there was nothing there... He came to a stop. He raised his eyes. Clenched a fist. Then he turned to Randle.

'Give them back!' he said.

'What?' said Randle. 'What are you on about?'

'I'll say this once and only once. Give them back now, or by heaven I'll...' said a red-faced Wings.

Dirk got up and opened the door for them.

'You blithering imbecile, what are you on about now?' said Randle, which only enraged Wings further.

Gently, Dirk ushered Randle out into the corridor. Wings followed. 'Damn you for a thieving devil, Randle, I know it was you – who else would it be?'

'By Jove, Wings, you've really lost it this time, haven't you!' said Randle as Dirk softly shut the door.

'Why, you..!' and then there was a crash, a bang, and a lot of shouting. Dirk couldn't control himself any more and burst out laughing. He opened the cupboard door, and there was Skinrash, stuffing his face with wine gums, and grinning up at Dirk happily.

'That went well, your Dirkness,' said Skinrash. 'Num, num, num!'

'Leave some black ones for me, you little green gobber,' said Dirk, patting him on the head., though on second thoughts, he probably shouldn't eat anything that had been handled by Skinrash. And he'd have to wash the hand that had done the patting.

# *Mrs Purejoie's Surprise*

Dirk left Skinrash to his face stuffing, and called in Dave the Storm Crow from outside the window. It was carrying a message from the Darklands, as Dirk had hoped. The Dark Library's Deadly Poisons section was probably the best possible place you could go to find out about poison and Agrash had completed an in-depth analysis. The Black Hag's poison was called the 'Malefic Taint' and various ingredients were involved – principally Black Oleander, Orcsbane (both only grew in the Darklands), Nightshade and Hemlock (which also grew on Earth). All of these ingredients were to be found in a little bottle strapped to Dave's leg. Agrash warned against touching any of them directly. 'Andel wiv care' had been daubed on it in crude Goblin writing.

Dirk put a hand to his chin and smiled. It would

have been hard to work out how to create an antidote back in his Alchemical Lab in the Iron Tower, but here on Earth? Even the school chemistry lab was leagues ahead of his, and the amount of information about how to make antidotes and antitoxins just on the internet alone, freely there for all to see, would make the job almost easy.

Well, provided you were an evil genius like him, of course! Without thinking, Dirk put his hands together and let rip with one of his trademark Evil Laughs.

'MWAH, HAH, HAH!'

'Oh do be quiet, Dirk,' said Mrs Purejoie from just outside the door. 'Anyway, would you open up please, your washing's done.'

'Excellent, my minion,' said Dirk, as he rose to his feet. 'It is good that you have brought my washing. When I conquer all, at least it will be in a nice clean shirt.'

'Yes, yes, very funny,' said Mrs Purejoie as she came into the room, arms full of Dirk's clothes. 'It took ages to get that nasty green stuff out of your dressing gown – I do wish you'd be more careful, Dirkikins.'

Mrs Purejoie dumped the clothes on his bed, turned and reached for the cupboard door. Dirk eyes widened with horror. Of course, she was going to hang everything up in the cupboard! Before he could say a word, she had yanked the door open...

To see Skinrash, frozen in fright, warty hand halfway up to his mouth, about to pop another wine gum in, eyes swivelled up in shock at the sight of her, face a mask of caught-in-the-act Goblin guilt.

Mrs Purejoie blinked in astonishment. Then she simply slumped to the floor in a dead faint.

Dirk stared at the body on the floor for a moment, thinking furiously.

'Quick, Skinrash,' he barked, 'under the bed with you, now!'

'Yes, Master,' said Skinrash, darting past the prone Purejoie and into the darkness beneath the bed.

'Don't come out, and whatever you do don't make a sound! Not even a single wine gum slurp! I mean it, I really Dark Lord mean it, you understand?!'

'Yes, Master,' said a cowed Skinrash.

'Jack, Jack!' Dirk shouted. 'Hilary's fainted!'

Seconds later, Dr Jack came running into the room.

'Hilary!' he gasped as he knelt down behind her. Dirk stepped back and folded his arms, observing. Dr Jack was instinctively doing the doctor thing, checking her pulse, lifting up her eyelids. Tenderly he picked her up and laid her on the bed.

Dirk frowned. He had to admit, they clearly loved each other. Also, they'd been good to him, never hit him, tortured him, tried to kill him with a sword, chain him up, burn him out of his home, throw holy water in his face or hire assassins to hunt him down and kill him. None of that.

'She just fainted, Jack,' said Dirk. 'Maybe she's tired, not eating properly with that church charity thing she keeps going on about that's been taking up all her time. And carrying all that washing, it's very heavy.'

Mrs Purejoie began to whimper a little.

'Hilary, can you hear me?' said Jack.

'I'll put the clothes away,' said Dirk. 'We don't want to overwork her, she needs rest, right? Or is there something else I can do – anything? I want to help.'

'No, that's fine, Dirk, thank you, you're a

good boy, you really are,' said Jack as he stroked Mrs Purejoie's brow.

Dirk grinned a bit at that. True, he was laying it on, but actually...you couldn't say that he *loved* the Purejoies, or even liked them that much, but he certainly didn't wish them any harm. Well, perhaps he liked them a little. When they weren't actually around, that is. You know, that sort of thing.

Mrs Purejoie came to – and shrieked! 'Argh! There's a...a thing! A thing in the cupboard!'

'A thing? What do you mean?' said Jack.

'A...creaturey thing, like one of those Goblins – a Goblin eating wine gums in the cupboard!' she wailed.

'What...' said Jack, turning to look at the cupboard. Dirk looked at Jack, a sympathetic expression on his face. He opened the cupboard door and pointed at its empty bareness.

''Fraid not,' he said, shaking his head.

Jack looked back. 'It's some kind of hallucination, dear, just like the last time with the lenses.'

'No! No, I saw it, in the cupboard,' she said.

'Now, now, my love. A Goblin, for a start... But eating wine gums? Really?' said Jack.

Mrs Purejoie wrinkled her brow. Then her face fell. 'Yes, yes, of course...' She looked up at her husband, her face uncertain and fearful. 'Do you think...do you think I'm going mad, maybe losing my mind?'

'No, no, dear, of course not,' said Dr Jack tenderly. 'You're probably overworked and overtired, making you see things. You'll be fine, I'm sure!'

'But why a Goblin?' she said.

Jack flicked a glance at Dirk. 'Well, you know... the room you're in...'

Mrs Purejoie looked at Dirk and then around the room – at the black, skull-covered curtains, the black, skull-covered bedspread, the chair and table carved with strange runes, the books and encyclopaedias on electronics, science, war, conquest and torture, Dirk's creepy phone and the rest.

'Right,' she said, understanding dawning on her face, 'that sort of makes sense, doesn't it?'

Dirk folded his arms. Nice, he thought to himself. But then he shrugged. He had to admit, they had a point.

'Quite. And don't worry, darling, I'll look after

you, do some tests,' said Dr Jack. Mrs Purejoie sat up, and, like the Trojan mother she was, reached for the clothes to hang them up.

'No, let me. You've had a terrible shock, you should probably go to bed and get some rest,' said Dirk, all kindness and care. Hilary smiled at him, put a hand to his cheek. Dirk began putting the clothes away, trying to be the dutiful son.

'Thank you, dear,' she said.

Suddenly, there was a low rush of sound, like the faint trickle of a stream and a terrible, noxious stench filled the room.

Goblin fart! thought Dirk to himself, as his face wrinkled up in disgust.

Mrs Purejoie actually went green. Dr Jack gagged.

Jack glared at Dirk. Dirk shook his head ever so slightly and nodded at Mrs Purejoie, who didn't look at anyone. In fact, it looked like she was going to faint again. Jack's jaw dropped as he stared at his wife.

'Wow, she really isn't well, is she?' he said. Then, quickly, he helped her up and hurried her out of the room, leaving Dirk to choke in a miasma of Goblin-gut vileness.

'Skinrash, you little...' muttered Dirk under his breath as he headed for the window, feeling quite nauseous himself. He leaned out and sucked in great gasps of clean fresh air. Poor Mrs Purejoie. Because of him, she'd seen a vision of a strange tower of evil in a dark land, and then a Goblin from another world, who promptly gassed her – and she'd got the blame for all of it. And now Jack would probably put her through a battery of pointless tests. Still, she'd recover.

He hoped.

'Anyway, she shouldn't have called me Dirkikins, eh, Skinrash?' said Dirk.

~~November 27th, 2013~~ Rip-out-their-hearts 27th

*Success! It's complicated, and time consuming, but I have managed to make some antidote. Not much, mind, but it is a start. In other news, Christopher has to do extra household chores for lying about the cake.*

*'Eat it, Christopher!' I said to him, which I thought was quite a good joke, but he didn't seem to agree. He's been very tetchy recently.*

*I've also had an interesting idea that might*

*delay or slow down Hasdruban long enough for
me to make more antidote.*

~~November 28th, 2013~~ Rip-out-their-hearts 28th
*I'm in for it now! Just got feedback from old
Battleaxe the English teacher on the last bit
of homework I did... Or more accurately, that
my minion Skinrash did for me. The little...
I mean, what was I thinking? They're calling
it 'gross insubordination' or some such and I
have to see the headmaster! He's sent a letter
to my parents saying I must attend his office
in a week's time. Interesting that it's a week,
though. Why not sooner? Because he thinks I
will be dead by then, that's why. Murdered by
the Black Hag.*

*I've attached that crazy Goblin's homework.
When, oh when will I get a truly reliable
minion?*

## Sentences – Test

Print

*Choose the best connective to join the following simple sentences.*

**1.** I pushed the door. It opened with a creak

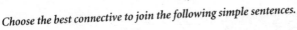

Smash it - hur, hur!

☐ *and*
☐ *but*
☐ *or*

**2.** It was a hot, bright day. The room was strangely cold.

☐ *and*
☐ *so*
☐ *but*

Burn table! Make room warm

**3.** The room was dark. I couldn't make out any objects apart from a huge armchair.

I like the dark, see fine...

☐ *but*
☐ *so*
☐ *although*

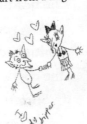

**4.** I took two or three steps into the room. I stopped.

☐ *then*
☐ *or*
☐ *although*

RAAAARGHH!

**5.** I heard a noise. My skin started tingling with fear.

☐ *and*
☐ *but*
☐ *or*

Aieee! Paladins! Run!

**6.** I could hear my own breathing. It sounded unnaturally loud.

☐ *so*
☐ *and*
☐ *or*

Farting sound louder! Hur hur!

Gorgon poo!

**7.** Something shot out of the shadows. It burst out of the room.

☐ *and*
☐ *or*
☐ *so*

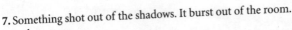

Goblinz attack, yaaaaahhh!

# Planting the Evidence

'All right, let's go over the plan one more time,' said Dirk. It was lunchtime at school and Chris, Sooz and Dirk were huddled together near the headmaster's study.

'We wait for the headmaster to leave his office,' continued Dirk, 'Chris stands watch at one end of the corridor, Sooz outside the door.'

Sooz nodded but Chris said, 'This is bonkers, it'll never work.'

'Worth a try, though,' said Dirk. 'I mean, look at it,' Dirk opened up his jacket and showed them... Skinrash's Goblin axe. The blade was covered in Darklands runes, and the handle strangely curved.

Sooz shook her head, 'I don't like it, Dirk,' she said.

'It's really serious, bringing that into school,' said Chris. 'If we get caught, we could be expelled – worse, we could go to jail!'

'Oh come on,' said Dirk, 'We've been through this before. And anyway, Hasdruban gave me the idea. It was him who made up stuff about me "making a gun"! OK, it's not a gun, it's a weapon from the Darklands, but still. It's only poetic justice to throw it back in his face!'

'Still, I don't like it either,' said Chris.

'Look, Hasdruban tried to kill me. With a sword. Now he's going to send a deadly assassin after me. He's "playing lardball" and so should we!'

Sooz grinned widely, and exchanged a look with Chris.

'What?' said Dirk.

'It's hardball, not lardball, Orcbrain!' said Chris, with a laugh.

'Orcbrain? How dare you!' shouted Dirk imperiously. 'My brain is far superior to that of an Orc! Indeed, I have commanded a hundred thousand of them before, in open war, across...'

'All right, all right, keep yer horns on,' said Chris, trying not to laugh any more (which would only make things worse, as he knew from bitter experience).

'Yeah, we need to concentrate!' said Sooz. 'Old

Whitey is playing hardball, you're right, Dirk. So we have to fight back too, OK, I get it.'

Dirk stared at her for a moment as he struggled to get his temper under control.

'Yes, yes, Chris, childish insults are neither here nor there. We must deal with the matter in hand,' said Dirk. 'So, the plan – after I put the Goblin axe in his study, we send some anonymous messages to the human police. It's a weapon in a school – they'll have to investigate. They'll find it and haul Hasdruban off for questioning. Sure, he'll probably get out of it – it's fake, planted there by the kids, blah, blah. They'll believe him too, I would think, but not for a few days at least! Give him a bit of headache, hold him up long enough for me to make more of the antidote. Got to be worth trying, right?'

'I guess,' said Sooz, not entirely convinced.

'Well, I've got nothing to lose. And we have to fight back, I can't just sit here and take hit after hit from Hasdruban – he's bound to succeed in the end. So, guys, please. Help me here. I need you!' said Dirk.

Chris sighed. Sooz raised her eyes. 'Yes, yes, all right then, we'll do it. I mean, we've got no choice – he's playing lardball and that, isn't he?'

she said, smiling at Chris.

Chris giggled.

'The harder you play, the fatter you get!' she added, rubbing her tummy. Both of them collapsed into gales of laughter.

Dirk folded his arms. '*Bah*, worthless humans!' he said, but that only made them laugh even more.

Dirk put his hands on his hips and glared at them. He was about to launch into a Dark Lord tirade but decided to try a different tack. So he said, 'Come on, guys, this is serious! My life is in danger here, real danger!'

That had the desired effect and shut them up.

'You're right,' said Sooz. 'I'm sorry, Dirk. Carry on with the plan.'

Dirk inclined his head, a silent thank you.

'All you have to do is keep watch, I'll do the rest,' said Dirk, just as the door to the headmaster's study opened, and out stepped Dr Hasdruban, white suit, cane, hat – the works. He was off to lunch.

'Quick,' hissed Dirk. 'Chris, you go to the end of the corridor, Sooz outside the study door! When you spot him coming back, Chris, signal Sooz. All she has to do is give me a shout, and I'll be out of there like a hat out of hell! Though really, I should only be a few minutes, anyway.'

'That's a bat out of...' began Sooz, 'Oh, never mind, let's go!'

Sooz and Chris nodded and headed off to their respective posts, although neither looked particularly happy about it. Dirk stepped up to the study door, made sure no one was around, and tried the door handle. It was unlocked. Why wouldn't it be?

Dirk stepped inside.

Hasdruban's study had been redecorated since he'd taken over from Grousammer. The walls were white, of course, and he'd had a big new desk put in, of heavy, burnished oak. Behind it was a large, managerial office chair, more like a throne than anything else. In front of the desk was another much smaller chair. It looked like it was bolted to the floor, as well. Newly installed too. Visitors would sit there, ready to be intimidated by the headmaster on his great throne. Standard practice for megalomaniacal overlords. And Dirk should know...

On the walls were various photos of Hasdruban, some obviously faked, as they showed him getting

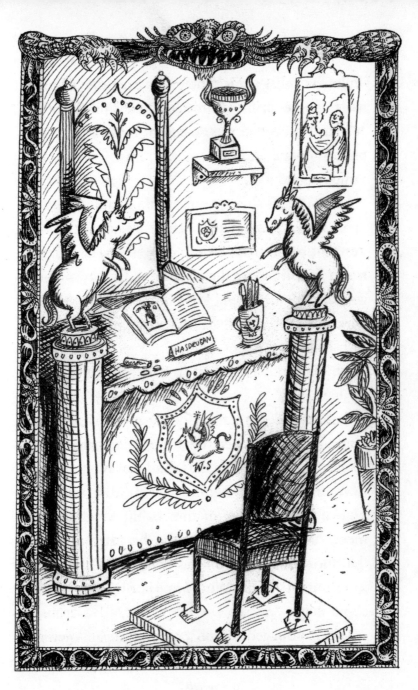

*A typical headmaster's study*

diplomas and awards. There was even one of him meeting the Prime Minister. Dirk smiled wryly at that. Hasdruban was so full of himself, he even photoshopped stuff to make himself look big! Puffed up old fool.

Dirk stepped smartly up to a filing cabinet, slid it open, wiped the goblin axe clean, and put it inside. Best not to put it in a desk drawer, as Hasdruban might find it before the police did. Dirk turned to go. He knew he should leave immediately but...but Dirk was Dirk, and there was a throne nearby. His arch-enemy's throne.

He stepped over and sat in the great white office throne.

He looked down at the desk. Hasdruban had some kind of magazine open. What was he reading...? An article, it seemed. About the founder of Whiteshields town, a certain Sir Ratum Swinefield. There was a great bronze statue of him in the Whiteshields memorial gardens. Apparently the marble plinth that the statue rested on was hollow and his bones were buried inside. Why was Hasdruban reading about that?

Dirk shrugged. Probably nothing. Anyway,

he'd better get on. But first...

'Detention, Lloyd!' said Dirk in his best Hasdruban voice. 'And you too, Purejoie, and also you, Susan Black!'

As he said this he pointed around the room imperiously as if handing out punishments willy-nilly at school assembly.

'And you, and you, in fact that whole class! No, wait, the whole school! The whole school is in detention, including the teachers! Eternal Detention for all!'

He began to laugh at his own joke, giggling like a madman. But then he noticed something odd. Something just under the desktop.

A button.

Dirk examined it closely. How odd. An alarm? Or something else? Dirk, curiosity piqued, reached for the button but at the last second he paused. What if it was an alarm, and brought teachers running? Or worse, even? Still, if it was, he'd have time to make a run for it....

Dirk couldn't help himself, he had to know. He hit the button.

Suddenly, the chair on the other side of the desk

disappeared from view with a loud clanking sound! Dirk looked over – the chair was fixed to a trap door that had opened over a pit below.

Dirk burst out laughing – a pit trap? How 'old skool' could you get? But then his laughter died, for at the bottom of the pit were several nasty-looking sharpened wooden stakes. Whoever fell down that pit would be impaled horribly. Death was certain. Dirk frowned. So this was what Hasdruban had planned for him, was it? He had to see the headmaster next week, because of Skinrash's hopeless homework effort – assuming he survived the Black Hag, that was! He'd have come in here, sat down...and then... that would've have been the end of Dirk!

'Well, we'll see about that,' said Dirk out loud. He hit the button and the trap door and the chair came back up again with a loud click. Then, as quick as he could, he set about rewiring the electrics so that instead of opening the trap door, it would short out and give Hasdruban sitting on the office throne a bit of an electric shock. Not enough to kill him, there wasn't the power to do that, but enough to give him a nasty shock! Either way, it would be fun, just to see his face.

He was halfway through the job when Sooz hissed at him from outside.

'What are you doing in there, Dirk? It's nearly two o'clock!'

'I need more time,' said Dirk.

'There is no more time! We have to go to lessons – now!' said Sooz.

'Just a few more minutes,' said Dirk.

'Come on, get out…wait, here comes old Battleaxe, we've got to go, sorry, Dirk!'

'OK, go, go, I'm almost there.'

But Sooz didn't hear him. She'd been shooed off to class by Mrs Batelakes, the English teacher.

After a few more minutes, Dirk was finished.

The thought of what would happen when Hasdruban pressed the button was so darkly delicious it deserved a 'Mwah, hah, hah' but that would be too noisy, so he contented himself with an evil cackle: 'Heh, heh, heh.'

Without warning, the study door swept open and Hasdruban walked in! It was all that Dirk could do to drop down out of sight into the well of the desk. He just managed it without being seen.

Hasdruban walked around the desk and sat down.

His feet shot forward, almost kicking Dirk, where he was huddled in the corner of the desk well. But it was a big desk, and Dirk was small enough to avoid Hasdruban's legs and feet. He stared at Hasdruban's shoes in fascination. Finely crafted white leather brogues. With pale grey laces.

Hasdruban crossed his feet. Dirk could hear paper rustling. And humming. A song Dirk recognised, a centuries old war song from the Darklands, sung by the Paladins of the Whiteshields, about how many Orcs they would kill in battle, and how they'd burn down the Iron Tower. Then they'd kill the Dark Lord and mount his great horns over the barracks' door as a trophy.

What was it called? Oh yes, 'The Dark Lord's Demise'. The Paladins would often sing the chorus over and over again at the end. 'Reprise the Demise', they called it, like a kind of ritual drinking song.

*Bah*, fanciful nonsense, thought Dirk to himself. And was that all Hasdruban thought about, his destruction? He was obsessed, completely obsessed!

Dirk began to stare at Hasdruban's shoelaces. It would be so easy to undo them, then tie them together. Dirk put a hand to his mouth, stifling the naughty schoolboy giggle that was trying to burst up out of him. Imagine it! Hasdruban trying to get up and falling over... But when he did imagine it, he could see Hasdruban lying on the floor, staring straight at Dirk hiding under his desk...that soon put paid to his giggles. Hasdruban still had his sword cane with him, after all.

Suddenly the telephone rang. The headmaster jerked in his chair, startled by the ringing.

'I hate telephones,' he muttered under his breath, before picking it up and saying, 'Hasdruban the White... I mean, the headmaster! This is the headmaster speaking.'

A few seconds passed.

'What do you mean, there's a fire in the music room? Who is this?' said Hasdruban.

Dirk could hear a faint tinny sound of a raised voice on the other end of the phone.

'All right, all right – I don't know who you are, young lady, but if this is a schoolgirl prank, I will find you, and you *will* be punished!' said Hasdruban.

Dirk smiled. Sooz on the phone, for sure. She was ace!

Hasdruban slammed the phone down, leaped to

his feet and hurried out of his office.

Dirk sighed with relief. He eased his way out, opened the door, and peeked into the corridor. The coast was clear...quickly he hurried off to class. He was going to be late, and would probably get in trouble for it (again) but it was worth it!

Dirk's heart soared. He really felt as if he'd turned the tables on Hasdruban for once, what with the axe planted and his nasty little pit trap set up to backfire on him! As he approached old Battleaxe's class room, he just couldn't help himself and he had to pause, put his fingers together and let out a loud,

'MWAH, HAH, HAH!'

The door to English class opened and out leaned old Battleaxe, Mrs Batelakes.

'Ah, there you are, Dirk. Now stop that, and get in here, you naughty boy!'

# DermatoGlyphs

November 29th, 2013 Rip-out-their-hearts 29th
*Curses, foiled again! We fired off some
anonymous letters and emails to the police,
but it seems Hasdruban found the goblin axe
almost straight away and he handed it in. Then
they got the emails and letters! Now it really
looks like a set-up.*

*Which it was of course, but still, it is
frustrating!*

The next day, Dirk, Sooz and Chris went to school
as normal. As they walked through the main door,
they could see the headmaster up ahead, leaning
against the wall in a manner that Dirk could only
describe as 'sarcastic nonchalance'.

He nodded at the three of them as if he knew
exactly what they'd been up to.

'Good morning, children,' said the headmaster with a smile of purest insincerity.

'Good morning,' said the three kids together, the very model of dutiful schoolchildren, smiling back at him. Only their eyes betrayed their true feelings.

'In there please, Dirk,' said Hasdruban, pointing at the Reception offices. 'The police want to talk to you.'

Dirk frowned. 'The police? What lies have you been telling them this time?'

'Me! Not a thing. It's nothing to do with me,' said the headmaster.

'Yeah, right!' said Sooz, 'You expect us to believe that?'

'I find an axe in my study. I hand it in. The police are investigating. They need no prompting from me to work out the likely culprit, oh no!' said Hasdruban.

Dirk narrowed his eyes. 'Oh, really?' he said.

The headmaster leaned forward and hissed aggressively, 'Yes, really! You think I'd call them in? To do what? Lock you up? Expel you? *Bah* – they're next to useless, with their rights and rules and rehabilitations. I don't want you locked up, you spawn of hell, I want you dead!'

Dirk stared up at the headmaster defiantly, a cutting retort ready on his lips, but Sooz got in there before him.

'You're mad, and bad and we won't let you, never, ever!' said Sooz stamping her foot.

Dirk smiled at that. Hasdruban leaned back, folded his arms. 'See what you've become, Dark One? A pitiful wretch hiding behind the skirts of a little schoolgirl. Hah!'

The door to Reception opened and out leaned a policeman, quite a high-ranking one at that, by the look of him.

'Dirk Lloyd?' he said. 'I'd like a word please, if you'll come this way.'

Dirk looked the policeman over. 'Yes, insignificant human, I think I can allow you to interview me,' he said, knowing full well he didn't have much choice, but still, he had to hold up appearances and everything. The policeman put his arms behind his back, and rocked on his heels, frowning. It was the sort of response he'd been expecting. He'd read Dirk's file, after all. But still, to be actually addressed like that by a kid was rather unnerving.

Before he stepped away, Dirk whispered to the headmaster. 'A schoolgirl, true, but also the Moon Queen, Wielder of the Great Ring, the Dark Lady, and Queen of the Darklands – and don't you forget it!'

Hasdruban frowned. He looked over at Sooz. She smiled back him. 'Put out that fire in the music room all right, did you, sir?' she said.

'*Bah*,' hissed the headmaster, turning away, 'To the Nine Hells with the lot of you!'

With that he walked away.

'Come on now, young fellow,' said the policeman, beckoning Dirk over. 'We've got a few questions we need to ask you, won't take long.'

Dirk followed the policeman into a back room where they normally processed new admissions. His foster father, Dr Purejoie was there, along with another police officer.

'Hi, Dirk,' said Dr Purejoie. 'Now, I'm sure this is just a formality, but the police need to...check some stuff. I'm sure it'll be fine.'

'I'm sure it will,' said Dirk, not in the least bit intimidated. He was a Dark Lord, after all.

'Sit down, Dirk,' said the first policeman, pointing

at a chair. 'I'm Detective Inspector Hughes, this is Constable Handwinkle...'

Dirk couldn't help himself, and he sniggered.

Constable Handwinkle glared at him.

Detective Inspector Hughes raised his eyes. 'Why don't you just change your name, Handwinkle, eh? This happens nearly every time, it's pointless!' he said.

Constable Handwinkle shrugged. 'Never!' she said under her breath. 'We've been Handwinkles for hundreds of years.'

'Well then,' said DI Hughes, 'just learn to put up with it. Anyway, enough of that. Now, Dirk, we need to talk about...well, a kind of axe that was found in the headmaster's study. Why did you put it there?'

'I didn't,' said Dirk. 'It wasn't me.'

Everyone stared at him for a moment. Dirk folded his arms.

'Come on now,' said the Detective Inspector. 'We have a report from your therapists that you'd cut yourself and tried to blame the headmaster, and then – well, a weird-looking weapon from *Lord of the Rings* or something appears in the headmaster's study. We have social work reports, fostering reports and much else, all about you Dirk and your behaviour. Don't tell me it's a coincidence!'

'Yeah,' said the other police officer. 'We've got you bang to rights, kid, just tell us what we want to know and we'll go easy on you!'

'Hah, what a pitiful attempt to intimidate me, Blandstinkle – pathetic!'

Constable Handwinkle looked like she was going to lose her temper, but DI Hughes put a hand on her shoulder, calming her down.

Classic good Orc, bad Orc routine, thought Dirk to himself. Fools! Didn't they know who he was?

'Let's all keep this calm, shall we? Although, she's right, isn't she, Dirk? I mean, you only have to look at the evidence!' said DI Hughes.

'The evidence?' retorted Dirk. 'What evidence? It's drivel, all rumour and gossip! You have no proof of any of this, have you? Not one bit!' said Dirk imperiously. 'You think you can threaten me? ME, the Great Dirk! *Bah*, you fools – I've been through far worse than you can possibly imagine, your petty accusations are nothing to me!'

The three adults stared at him, completely thrown off balance.

'Told you,' said Dr Purejoie.

Detective Inspector Hughes glanced over at Dr Jack, and then back at Dirk.

'Well then,' he said. 'You won't mind if we fingerprint you then?' – expecting Dirk to panic a bit at that, but of course he didn't.

'Not at all,' said Dirk, uncrossing his arms. 'Not at all.' But inside he was thinking furiously. Had he made sure the Goblin axe was fingerprint free? Actually, he had, he'd wiped it clean – of course he had! He was fastidious about that sort of thing, as every great villainous mastermind should be.

'Fingerprint away,' he said, putting out his hand.

They brought out a fingerprinting kit, put each of Dirk's fingers of his right hand into the ink, and pressed them onto a piece of paper. Inspector Hughes stared at Dirk, as he sprinkled dust over the ink to dry it off. Dirk gave him a grin. The Inspector's jaw dropped.

'That grin... It's like...like...' started Inspector Hughes.

'The Fetbury Filleter...' finished the other police officer.

'What, the notorious serial killer?' said Dr Jack.

'The very same,' said the Detective Inspector, staring at Dirk in horror.

Dirk, however, hadn't really noticed the exchange. He was staring in fascination at the fingerprints. *His* fingerprints. None of the others had noticed, and it looked like they weren't going to, distracted by his grin as they were. Detective Inspector Hughes folded the prints away. Anyway, why would they give them more than a cursory examination? Forensic experts would be examining them in detail later. So they had missed what Dirk had seen.

His prints came out like this...

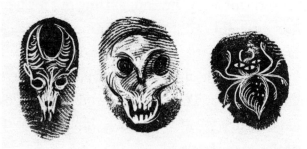

'Well, I suppose that's that, for now,' said Inspector Hughes. 'Thank you for your...cooperation. You may go.'

'OK, Dirk, off to class with you,' said Dr Jack.

Dirk rose up and headed for the door. He began

to think about what would happen when they checked his prints against any they found on the Goblin axe. For a start, if they found any, they'd probably be Hasdruban's. But when they looked at his...

They'd be confused, to say the least. Either Dirk was some kind of mutant freak or a some kind of supervillain genius. Or maybe they'd blame Inspector Hughes! As Dirk stepped out of the door, he began to laugh out loud.

'MWAH, HAH, HAH!'

Inside the admissions room, the three adults exchanged worried glances.

# The Battle of Swinefield

It was early evening, on a cold November's night. A damp mist filled the air, chilling the bones of any mortal foolish enough to venture out. In Whiteshields Memorial Gardens stood the statue of one of the great Victorian philanthropists of that age, the founding father of Whiteshields town, Sir Ratum Swinefield. The bronze figure of Sir Ratum, dressed in classical Greek clothing, holding an architect's set square in one hand, and a large white shield in the other, was pitted with verdigris and covered in bird...stuff.

Neglected. Forgotten.

It rested on a massive marble plinth. Latin words carved onto the plinth declaimed his greatness to all. Unfortunately, hardly anyone could read Latin anymore, so who knew what it said? And hardly anyone ever came to the gardens – or Swinefield, as the locals called them – for they were no longer kept up as gardens and the town's one way system made it difficult to get to, and there was nowhere to park.

Nevertheless, despite the weather and its remoteness, two slight figures approached the statue, wrapped up in coats and scarves – Sooz and Christopher. They loitered nearby, looking around.

'Where is he?' said Sooz.

'Dunno, but he definitely texted you?' asked Chris.

'Yeah. He said to be here at six,' said Sooz checking the time on her mobile phone.

'Well, he's usually pretty punctual,' said Chris.

'Yeah,' said Sooz.

'By the way, have I shown you this yet?' said Christopher, and he pulled out a metal flask from his pocket. It was all black, with a skull and cross bones on the front. Underneath the skull the words 'The Dark Lord' were inscribed.

'Hah, that's cool!' said Sooz, as she took the flask to examine it.

'I got it online – they write what you want on it,' said Chris.

'Brill,' said Sooz, handing it back. 'Present for Dirk, right?'

'Yeah, thought I'd...put something in it,' said Chris, hesitantly.

Sooz said, 'Well, make sure whatever it is that it's black – you know, like blackcurrant or black tea or cola or something.'

'Oh yeah, it'll be black all right!' said Chris.

'When are you going to give it to him, dude?' said Sooz.

'Dunno yet, later. A surprise for when we get Hasdruban out of the way or something, so don't mention it!' said Chris.

'Right...oh, look here he comes,' said Sooz, 'put it away!' Chris hurriedly stashed the flask in a pocket.

'Hi, guys,' said Dirk, as he drew near through the misty cold. 'What did you want, Sooz?' He too was dressed in a coat and scarf. Black, of course.

Sooz frowned. 'What did I want? You texted me, all mysterious and that – and why here?'

Dirk seem surprised. 'But I didn't... I mean, it was you – you texted me!'

'No, no, you said meet us here, and that I should tell Chris....'

Dirk's eyes widened as realisation dawned – the magazine on Hasdruban's desk. Of course!

'It's a trap!' he shouted.

Suddenly, one side of Sir Ratum Swinefield's plinth split open with a shattering crack and out of the dark, hollow interior leaped a black figure! A figure dressed in long, ragged black lace, with a strange, cobwebbed black headdress, a ripped up black veil, and arm length tattered black velvet gloves. Her fingers ended in long, iron talons dripping with venom.

'The Black Hag!' screamed Dirk. Everyone took an involuntary step back, faces white with shock and fear.

She was small – about the same size as Dirk, but her long taloned nails and strange headgear made her look bigger. She fixed her pale all-white eyes upon Dirk.

'All shall mourn!' she said in a voice like dry sand pouring into a bowl, followed by, 'Dieeee!', as she sprang forward like a pouncing spider, swiping her claws at Dirk.

Dirk had to drop backwards onto the ground to avoid the envenomed talons.

The Black Hag stepped forward, straddling Dirk's prone body. He raised his arms up protectively –

though they were no protection at all, as she had only to scratch him to kill him.

Chris and Sooz snapped out of their shock. They darted in, trying to knock the Lady Grieve away from Dirk.

The Black Hag swayed from side to side, slashing at them.

'Nooo!' said Dirk, 'Don't let her touch you, not even the slightest scratch! Get back, get back!'

Sooz and Chris dodged aside.

'Don't worry, my pretties, your turn will come,' hissed the Black Hag as she turned her attention to the small boy beneath her, who was trying desperately to scramble away, heels slipping on the wet grass.

'Run, you two, run!' said Dirk to Sooz and Chris.

The Black Hag put a dirty bare foot on Dirk's chest, pinning him in place. 'My, aren't we the hero – Hasdruban was right, you aren't the Dark One I knew of old,' she said, raising her taloned hands into the air. 'Not that I care either way.'

Sooz and Christopher hesitated, half in fear, half in guilt, not wanting to leave Dirk on his own, but knowing that one touch from those claws and they were dead. A tear sprang to Sooz's eye. When the chips were down, when they were in real danger, Dirk was sacrificing himself for them. Or that's what she and Christopher thought. But they didn't know what Dirk knew – that he had a single dose of antidote in his pocket. That was all he'd had time to make.

'I mean it, flee, you fools, flee,' said Dirk, as he reached into his pocket. All he had to do was take the pain, pretend to be dead and then quaff the antidote...assuming she didn't rip his throat open with those iron talons just to be sure, or the poison didn't kill him in an instant. Her claws came down. Dirk closed his eyes. Was this it?

'No!' cried Sooz, and she leapt forward.

Suddenly the Black Hag froze, her white, pallid eyes staring at something nearby.

'YOU!' she hissed hoarsely, and she stepped forward over Dirk, as if she'd just forgotten he was there. Dirk twisted on the ground to see what had distracted her, Sooz crashing down beside him, Chris a few moments behind.

Ahead out of the wispy fog came a figure, pale and wan, dressed in billowing white robes – the

White Witch!

Dirk's heart sank. 'How can we fight both of them?' he said.

'Wait,' said Sooz. 'Look!'

The Black Hag and the White Witch began to circle each other, the Black Hag holding her arms wide, talons spread like poisoned branches of death, the White Witch holding only a flimsy dagger.

'My Eternal Enemy,' rasped the Black Hag. The White Witch nodded at her.

'Of course,' said Dirk, getting to his feet. 'They are sworn enemies, deadly foes, each the mirror of the Light and the Dark – a thousand years of bitter enmity!'

The Black Hag began to smile, revealing crooked black teeth. 'But this time, you have no magic, no potions, no holy fires,' she said in a voice like a dusty tomb. 'There is only the Malefic Taint.'

She darted forward, scything at the White Witch, who hopped backwards.

Dirk frowned. This wasn't looking good for the White Witch. She was taller and stronger than the Black Hag, but actual hand to hand combat wasn't her thing, whereas the Black Hag was in her element

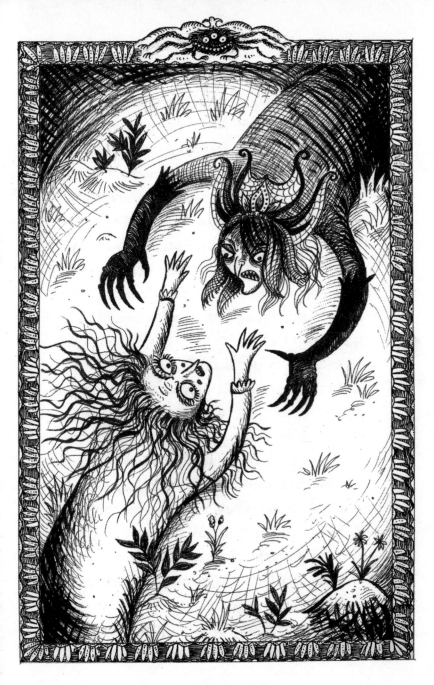

*Witch vs Hag, Round One!*

and none of the White Witch's magic would work here on Earth. And the Hag was fast. Anyway, what was the White Witch doing here? Why did she come? The Black Hag was doing Hasdruban's bidding, after all.

'We'd better get out of here,' said Chris. 'Now!'

'Yeah,' said Sooz, 'this isn't our fight!'

'Wait,' said Dirk, 'something doesn't add up.'

The White Witch lunged with her dagger. Lady Grieve hopped back and hacked down at her arm with the talons. The Witch jerked her hand back just in time.

'What shall we do?' said Chris.

'I dunno,' said Dirk, 'Maybe intervene, tip the odds...'

'Yeah, but on whose side?' said Sooz.

Dirk shrugged. 'That is the question!' he said.

The Black Hag gave a hoarse wail, leaped forward and swiped at the Witch, who gave ground rapidly. Dirk frowned. The White Witch was backing away – towards Dirk and Chris and Sooz. Was she trying to lead the Black Hag to them? Why turn up at all then? Or...what was going on?

The Black Hag darted forward, and swiped low

at the Witch's legs – she dodged to the side – but a talon scratched her, ever so lightly, on the calf. Even that slight scratch left an inflamed mark. The White Witch grimaced in pain.

The Black Hag hissed in triumph. Most ordinary folk would already be paralysed and dying but the White Witch was resistant to the Black Hag's poison. Still, it was having an effect. Several hits from the Black Hag would probably do the trick.

'Oh how sweetly shall I mourn your death!' said the Lady Grieve.

The White Witch's face was screwed up in pain, but she still managed a defiant smile.

Then Dirk noticed something – it looked like a roll of wallpaper or a newspaper, but made of leather or something similar. The White Witch had let it fall nearby. Dirk snatched it up.

'Aha!' he said, 'it's a rolled up Hole.'

'What?' said Chris and Sooz together.

'A Magic Hole. Simply lay it on the ground like so...' said Dirk as he rolled it out in front of him. It settled onto the grass. And became a hole. A black hole of nothingness in the ground.

Sooz and Chris stared at it in astonishment.

'Whatever you do, do not step on it! It is a way between worlds – I'll bet Hasdruban and the Witch have a bunch of these saved up and are travelling back and forth! It explains a lot, actually.'

'But how do you know where you're going to end up?' said Sooz.

'Good question,' said Dirk, but he was suddenly interrupted by a strange wailing, like some kind of animal braying in pain. The three of them stared in astonishment, for the White Witch had made that noise. She never made a sound, normally. But this time she'd been scratched badly on the shoulder.

'Should we use the Hole?' said Chris.

'No, no, I think the White Witch dropped it on purpose,' said Dirk.

Just then the Black Hag began to cackle, like a faerie tale witch, a high-pitched, horrible, hideous cackling. In fact, she was cackling so much she had to stop and catch her breath. The White Witch turned to look at Dirk. She saw that he'd unfurled the Hole, and she gave him a wan smile.

'But why?' said Sooz, as the White Witch began to back away to the Hole.

'I think she's going to try and get the Black Hag

to step through it,' said Dirk.

'Really? She's going to save you?' said Chris.

'Yup. She's finally seen the light. Or should I say the dark?'

Sooz frowned. 'Are you sure? I mean, really sure?'

'Nope, not entirely. But I think we're about to find out!'

The White Witch was only inches from the Hole. Suddenly, she jumped forward, and wrapped her arms around the Black Hag, who gasped in surprise.

'You fool,' rasped the Hag, 'I have you now!'

The White Witch picked her up, and turned, just as the Black Hag raked her talons down her back, leaving long bloody scratches. The White Witch moaned in agony, but now she had the Hag over the Hole.

The Hag looked down. 'No!' she said, as the White Witch let go. The Black Hag fell into the blackness.

'The Caverns of Grief!' shrieked the Black Hag at the last moment, and then suddenly she was gone.

'Of course – that's how you get to where you want to go!' said Dirk, 'You have to shout out your destination.'

Dirk turned to the White Witch. 'Pretty cool

Magic Hole. But expensive, really expensive – Hasdruban must have pulled out all the stops to get me, eh?'

The White Witch nodded. And sank to her knees. Her skin, usually pale and almost translucent, was blotchy and pink. Black lines began to trace their way across her face. She was dying.

The Magic Hole began to shimmer and ripple, and then suddenly it winked out of existence with a black flash.

'But why?' said Dirk. 'Why sacrifice yourself for me?'

She pointed at Chris and Sooz, as if to say, 'Typical, it's not just you.' Then she sank back onto the grass, breathing hoarsely. She reached into a pocket and handed Dirk a black card, covered in white writing.

*Can the Dark Lord be forgiven? Can he be redeemed? Perhaps. But his friends are innocent and a boy can be redeemed. Nor could I stand by whilst a boy – a strange boy, yes, but a boy nevertheless – is murdered foully by the Black Hag. Hasdruban has been blinded by his lust for justice, he has become that which he seeks to destroy. So I have made my choice and I die, but I am still of the light, I am still a White Witch, I am uncorrupted, I am pure, I have done my duty.*

'Wow,' said Dirk, 'that's one hell of a speech for you, Dumpsy Deary!' said Dirk. The White Witch smiled wanly up at Dirk, her skin beginning to go black with poison. He handed the note to Sooz who read it, and handed it on to Chris.

Sooz looked down at the Witch. 'We can't let her die,' she said.

Dirk nodded, and he reached for the small bottle in his pocket. Dirk leaned over the Witch. She looked up at him with her pale, grey eyes, the light in them slowly fading. Dirk poured the contents into her mouth.

'Antidote, Miss Deary,' he said, 'to the Malefic Taint – you're going to live!'

The White Witch's eyes widened in surprise.

'Nobody kills the Dark Lord's nanny, nobody!' said Dirk loudly.

# An Antidote to White Wizards?

The White Witch lay on her back, gasping for air. Dirk had administered the medicine, but was it going to work? Sure, the White Witch was resistant to the Malefic Taint but she'd taken a massive dose of venom, and Dirk hadn't been able to test the antidote properly.

Sooz reached forward, and held the Witch's hand. Slowly, ever so slowly, the Witch's breathing began to steady. The black lines began to fade and her skin slowly returned to normal.

After a while, the White Witch sat up, looking up at Dirk. She smiled at him. An unexpected turn of events, thought Dirk to himself.

'Well, what now then?' he said. The Witch drew out her black paper and her white pen and began scribbling furiously.

*I shall return home and get well. Never will I serve*
*Hasdruban again. I have two Magic Holes left,*
*one I will use, the other I gift to you. Use it wisely.*
*Remember this: the tears of the Lady Grieve, when*
*consumed, fill the drinker's heart with Empathy.*
*Those who hate will understand the minds of their*
*enemies and see them in a new light. Perhaps if you*
*can get a tear and trick Hasdruban into drinking*
*it, he will see you for what you truly are and finally,*
*after all these years, the Light and the Dark, the*
*Black and the White, can have Peace.*

Dirk read her note, and passed it on to Sooz. The
Witch stood up.

'That'd be great!' said Sooz. 'Peace between the
Darklands and the Commonwealth, between Goblins
and humans. It's everything I was working for when I
was the Dark Queen.'

The White Witch put a hand to Sooz's face, as if to
say, 'I know, I understand now.'

Sooz smiled back at her. 'We have to do it, Dirk, we
have to try!' she said.

'All very well, but to get a tear...we'd have to travel to
the Caverns of Grief, defeat the Black Hag in her den,

on her own territory!' said Dirk.

The White Witch nodded and scribbled another note.

*Nobody said it was going to be easy.*

Dirk read it, and passed the note to Sooz. She laughed, past it on the Chris. Chris didn't bother to read it – he just threw it onto the floor, annoyed that he was the last in line as usual.

No one noticed.

The White Witch handed Dirk a rolled up Hole, and unfurled the other. She turned to Dirk, and held out a hand. Dirk shook it. The Witch nodded at Sooz and Christopher, pulled out what looked like an iPhone and then stepped onto the Hole, pressing a button on the phone as she did so.

A mechanical voice spoke from the phone. 'The Lair of the White Witch,' it said. She sank into the Hole and was gone.

~~November 29th, 2013~~ Rip-out-their-hearts 29th
*What a night! Still, I have some time before bed to work up another newsletter. Amazingly, I've had some real letters from some of my readers!*
*Issue three of the* Dark Times *available now!*

# THE DARK TIMES

Issue Three     Price: 5 Copper Christophers

*'Why is the Dark Lord always the bad guy? It's just not fair.'*
Dirk Lloyd

## Today's Horrorscope

~~Scorpio~~ *Deathsting* – You are one day older. This will continue, until eventually you will get even older, and older and then die, probably of old age.

~~Cancer~~ *Nastynip* – Today, a race of super powerful mutant ants will rise up and carry you off and feed you to their Queen. Possibly. Come to think of it, maybe not.

~~Pisces~~ *Stinkyfish* – Stuff will happen to you. Some of it will be good, some of it will be bad. Maybe even really good. Or really bad. Amazing, eh?

<u>*Virgo Good-for-sacrifices*</u> – Today you will read something called the *Dark Times*. It's true, isn't it? See, how good am I?

<u>*Taurus Bullocks*</u> – Today you will be abducted by aliens. You will wake up on their ship to find out all the aliens are dead, leaving you in charge of the space ship, trapped on the wrong side of the galaxy with only a damaged computer as a companion. How will you get home? Watch out for stowaways...

## Letters with the Aunt of Agony

Dear Aunt of Agony,
Grotty Grout put me in detention because my dog ate my homework and he didn't believe me! What can I do?
Rebecca Hern

*Dear Rebecca,*
*Your options are:*
*1: Give your dog a massive dose of laxative, get the homework and hand it in.*
*2: Offer to put your dog in detention instead of you.*

*3: Put Grotty Grout in a huge cauldron, cook him up and feed him to your dog.*
*4: Suck it up and do the detention.*
*Yours Sneeringly,*
*The Aunt of Agony*
*PS I don't believe you either.*

Dear Aunt of Agony,
Recently I was bitten by a strange glowing spider and now I seem to have developed spider-like abilities. I have grown several new eyes, and can spit super hard silk webbing, climb up walls and ceilings, jump huge distances and so on.
Unfortunately, I've also been shrunk down to the size of a spider.
Yours,
Paul Parker

*Dear Paul*
*You are doomed. Try not to get trodden on.*
*Yours Sneeringly,*
*The Aunt of Agony*

Dear Aunt of Agony,

I have managed to get the Hogweed, collected at the right time, and even the ground up bones of a murderer hung at a crossroads. Salt water too, that was easy obviously, but I am having trouble finding a bird called a Storm Crow.

Can you help?

Yours,

Laura Wibblebottom

*Dear Laura,*

*What the...? How in the Nine Hells did you get..?*

*Well, anyway. Umm... Storm Crow feathers – I think I can help you with that. PM me.*

*Yours Sneeringly,*

*The Aunt of Agony*

This issue of the *Dark Times* brought to you by the Great Dirk!

Yours Unfaithfully,

*I, the Dark Lord, Master of the Legions of Dread and Sorcerer Supreme, etc etc*

# Tears of Grief

Sunday, the first of December, in a clearing in a forest in Sussex, England. Several figures stand in a semi circle around a small boy, aged about thirteen years old. Two of the figures are of the same age. The other three are a tall human warrior, a horned and scaled winged demon and a Goblin. Typical Sussex crowd, really.

The small boy was telling the others what to do.

'So, mission name: The Tears of Grief! Ultimate goal – feed one of the Black Hag's tears to Hasdruban – he gets all sympathetic and nice, we make peace, everyone lives happily ever after.'

They all nodded, except for Rufino.

'One does not simply walk into the Caverns of Grief and take a tear,' he said.

'Indeed. But that's what we're going to do. So the plan is that we use a Magic Hole and all of us travel to the Caverns of Grief.'

'Well, at least we'll be going in force. Where are these Caverns, exactly?' said Rufino.

'In the Ash Mountains,' said Dirk.

'Where them Highland Orcs live?' said Skinrash.

'Yup, that's it. Not that far from home, in fact,' said Dirk.

'So, when it's all over, we go home easy?' said Gargon.

'Yes, that's the plan. We use a Magic Hole, and all of us go to the Caverns of Grief. We'll confront the Black Hag and demand a tear. Hopefully, she'll realise she's got no chance against all of us, and just hand one over – cry into a bottle or something.'

'Really? She'll give up just like that? I mean, one scratch from her and you're dead,' said Chris, 'She could take us all down!'

Dirk held up his hand, showing the ring on his finger. 'You forget, Chris, I'll have the Great Ring of Power, and it'll be working fine over there. Not to mention Gargon and Rufino, who are two of the greatest warriors in the Darklands, ever.'

Chris nodded at that. 'That's true. OK, I get it,' he said.

'Not to mention the antidote,' said Dirk.

'Antidote?' said Rufino.

'Yup, I have created an antidote to the Malefic Taint. As soon as I have made enough for each and every one of us to have a dose, we'll be able to start our great quest.'

'Huh, Dark Master is clever!' grated Gargon.

'You're a genius, your Braininess,' said Skinrash obsequiously.

'Yes, yes, enough of the flattery,' said Dirk.

'Really?' said Sooz.

Dirk gave her a look. She smiled back. 'OK, so chances are she'll just give us a tear, I can see that – Ring, Gargon, Goblin, Paladin etc. What then? Presumably Gargon, Rufino and Skinrash stay in the Darklands, the three of us kids come back home? How?'

'Well, that's something to think about,' said Dirk. 'We can come home, using the last Anathema Crystal. Or we could stay in the Darklands...'

Sooz frowned. 'All three of us?'

'Yeah,' said Dirk. 'You and I could be Dark Lord and Lady, we could live in the Iron Tower and rule, like I...I mean we! Like we were born to.'

'And you'd have the Ring of Power?' said Sooz.

Dirk stared at her for a moment. Rufino folded his arms, following the conversation with interest, as did Gargon. Skinrash meanwhile, was itching a buttock and looking at the birds in the trees, clearly bored.

'Yeah...' said Dirk. 'I'd have the Ring.'

'So it'd be like last time, you as the Dark Lord, me as...well...what exactly?' said Sooz.

'No, it wouldn't be like that! It'll be me, Dirk, just me, and...'

'What about me?' said Chris. 'How do I fit in then? General dogsbody and lackey, is that it?'

'General Dogsbody? Is that a title? Sure, you can be... Oh, I see... No, no, you'd be...whatever you want. Err...the Mouth of Dirk or something!'

'Meh, sounds like a lot of tosh to me. Last time all I got out of it was this scar,' said Christopher, fingering his cheek. 'Anyway, what about Hasdruban? He'll still be here, won't he?'

'Yes, true, but once we're in the Darklands, he'll go back to his White Tower, and it'll be much easier to face him in the Darklands with an army of Orcs and Goblins behind my back!'

'But much harder to feed him a tear,' said Sooz.

'And you think he's just going to go home, do you?' said Chris. 'What if he decides to kidnap my mum and

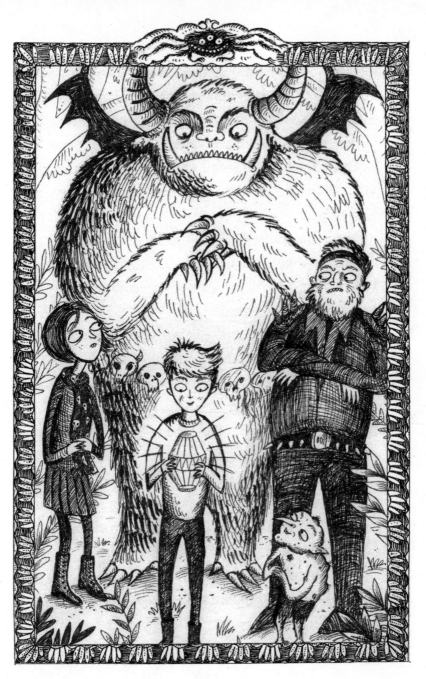

*Making plans after school*

dad, or Sooz's mum. Use them as hostages. Or some other nefarious plan while we're away?'

Dirk blinked. He was about to say, 'I hadn't thought of that...' but then thought better of it. Didn't want to let them know he'd missed a trick there. He frowned. Why hadn't he thought of that? It's what he would have done...

'He'd do it too,' said Sooz, 'he's that ruthless!'

'True, he would,' said Dirk. 'Of course he would, I knew that – I was just exploring possibilities – you know, options and such.'

'Well, definitely sounds like we'll have to come back here, deal with Hasdruban first,' said Sooz.

'But then we'll be marooned on Earth with no way to get home,' said Dirk.

'Your home, Dirk. We'll be where we belong,' said Chris.

'Anyway,' said Sooz, 'I'm sure we can work something out once the Hasdruban threat's been neutralised. You can get Agrash to get another Hole or something.'

'Yes, indeed. The sound is good,' said Dirk.

'No, that's "sounds good"...oh, forget it. How will you feed a tear to that madman, Hasdruban?' said Chris.

'Actually, I've got an idea for that,' said Dirk, 'But we have to get a tear first!' said Dirk.

'It is a plan that might even work,' said Rufino. 'One question, though: six of us have to go through that Magic Hole. One of them is seven foot tall with huge wings. Will we all fit in, and will it stay open long enough for us all to get through?'

'Good point,' said Dirk, 'And the truth is that I don't really know. Well, Gargon will fit, I know that – the Hole expands and contracts. But what I don't know is how long it will stay active. We'll have to take our chances.'

'We'd better work out who goes first then,' said Sooz.

'Yeah,' said Dirk, 'I thought me first – I'll have the Ring and I'm the most important.'

Chris and Sooz both folded their arms, brief flashes of irritation flitting across their faces. Dirk went on, oblivious, 'Then Gargon – he's the toughest, I'll need him on the other side, then Rufino, then Skinrash, then Sooz and then finally Chris.'

'Oh, so as usual I'm the least useful and the last to go. I mean, why bother? Why should I go at all?' said Chris angrily.

'You're my friend, Chris. I need people I can trust!' said Dirk.

'Oh please, you've got me last, you don't even need me – why pretend any more? You treat me like dirt, take me for granted all the time!' said Chris, his voice rising.

'Maybe he is right, best leave him behind,' said Rufino. 'No offence Christopher, your heart is true, but the Caverns are a dangerous place for an Earth boy.'

Christopher harrumphed angrily. 'Yeah, wouldn't want to be a burden,' he said. 'Anyway, what do you know about my heart?' he added, muttering under his breath.

'No!' said Dirk. 'I need you. Tell you what – here you are, Chris, here is the Anathema Crystal.' He reached into his pocket, drew out the crystal and handed it over. 'You are the Keeper of the Crystal, charged with making sure we all get back home to Earth safely!'

Rufino exchanged a look with Sooz. He didn't think this was such a good idea. Sooz shrugged. 'Actually, after the last time, I think it's a really good idea for Chris to have the crystal,' she said. 'Better than Dirk having it.'

Chris seemed a little mollified by that. He took the crystal from Dirk – a tad grudgingly, but he took it and placed it in his satchel.

'See!' said Dirk. 'Now you are extremely important

to the whole venture – so you have to go second, after me. Without you, no one gets home!'

'Are you sure about this, Dirk?' said Rufino. 'The Black Hag is deadly!'

'Don't forget, though – we'll have a dose of antidote each. And I know it works, we tested it on the White Witch, remember?'

'That's true,' said Sooz. 'It's not nearly as bad as it sounds.'

Skinrash piped up, 'Everyone gets some antidote? Even Goblins?'

'Yeah, even the Goblins,' said Dirk with a chuckle. 'OK, then. Is everyone set?'

'Suppose so,' said Chris.

'Yup, got it, dude,' said Sooz.

'Yes, your Superlativeness!' said Skinrash, though he didn't look too happy about it.

'Aye, your Dirkness,' said Rufino.

'Gargon get it, my Dark Lord!' he grated.

'Right then, Skinrash, Gargon and Rufino camp out here. Me, Chris and Sooz will return here on Monday night at 7 pm after school. I'll have enough antidote by then.'

## Local News

# 'ORC AXE' FOUND IN LOCAL SCHOOL

By our Education correspondent, Freda Lindquist

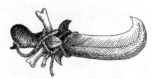

Dr Hasdruban, the headmaster of a local school, handed in a most extraordinary find yesterday - a replica fantastical axe! It was planted in his study, in an attempt to discredit him, he claims.

The officer investigating, Constable Carwyn Hughes, had this to say, 'It's more of a schoolboy prank than a criminal offence. I mean, the axe was hopelessly amateur-looking, of shoddy workmanship and as blunt as a spoon. Clearly knocked up in metalwork by one of the children.'

I then asked him this: 'Constable Hughes? Weren't you Detective Inspector Hughes only last week? What happened? Care to comment?'

'I'm not here to talk about that!' said Constable Hughes. 'Now get that microphone out of my face!'

---

~~December 1st 2013~~ Dirkmas 1st

*Shoddy workmanship? Amateur? How dare they! It's one of my best Goblin designs!*

# *The Helter Skelter of Doom*

D irk jumped into the glowing black hole in the
ground and yelled at the top of his voice, 'The
Caverns of Grief!'

In an instant, he was engulfed in total darkness.
He found himself rushing through some kind
of magical tube, like the ones in water parks – a
Helter Skelter of Doom. Strange faces and images
flashed by with shrieks and howls and horrific
screams. Phantasmal skeletal hands reached for
him, cobwebs brushed his face, and spectral heads
leered at him out of the dark. Fortunately for Dirk,
he was used to this sort of thing, and rather liked
impenetrable shadows filled with shrieking pale
skulls and ghostly faces. He began to think how
he could go about recreating the whole experience
as some kind of amusement park ride. The Dark

Lord's Helltour Skullter or something.

Suddenly, he popped out into bright sunlight and crashed onto a dusty, ash-covered slope. He sat up, a little dazed by his breakneck descent. He was on the side of a bone-white mountain, its stony surface bleached in the harsh light of the sun. It was dry and hot, and virtually nothing grew there. The air almost burned your lungs when you breathed it in.

Suddenly, a screaming boy crashed on top of him.

'Arrr...ow!' howled the boy.

'Get off me, you little earthling!' said Dirk.

'What, what,' said Chris, looking around in confusion. 'Wow, that was terrifying...'

Dirk looked up – his eyes widening in shock. 'Move, move,' he shouted, bundling himself and Christopher aside.

Just in time... A massive, winged, scaled and horned creature came crashing out of the sky to land in a great cloud of dust just where Chris and Dirk had been sitting.

'Roaaawrh!!!' bellowed Gargon. 'That was fun!'

'Yes, yes, all very well, Gargon, but get ready, here comes Rufino!' said Dirk. Above them, a tall figure came plummeting, his face white with shock.

Gargon was ready, though – he stood up smartly and caught Rufino in his arms.

For a moment, Rufino lay there, his arms around Gargon's neck, looking up at him like a baby.

'Awww, look, diddums,' said Chris in an exaggerated baby voice, glad to be distracted from the nightmare journey he'd just undergone. Dirk burst out laughing, his laughter echoing around the mountain side, a sound that probably hadn't been heard there in a thousand years or more.

The great demon and the mighty Paladin blinked at each other in embarrassment.

'Umm...you can put me down now,' said Rufino.

'Yeah, Gargon put you down, *now*!' gravelled the demon, pretty much dropping Rufino like a hot potato.

Dirk frowned. 'Wait a minute,' he said, 'who's next – Skinrash? He should have been here by now.'

'Could be the Hole has closed up,' said Chris. But then another figure appeared in the air above them, her face a mask of terror – Sooz!

'AAAAAArrgghgh!' she screamed.

Gargon stepped forward, and caught her neatly in his great arms, taking care not to scratch her with his taloned hands.

Sooz looked up at him.

'Thank you, Gargie,' she said, before resting her head against his mighty chest, taking a moment to get her breath back and to recover from the terrifying ghost train of a ride. Gargon looked down at her tenderly.

'That's all right, my Lady, Gargon happy to help,' he grated, an expression of tender care on his fanged visage. Well, probably – it was actually quite hard to tell what his expression was, unless you knew him well.

'So,' Dirk coughed. 'Back to the matter in hand. Where's Skinrash?'

Sooz got down out of Gargon's arms. 'Well, I watched him jump into the Hole all right, but then I think...maybe he got the words wrong.'

'By the Nine Hells, that could be dangerous! What did he say?'

'Umm...' hesitated Sooz.

'What? I mean, if he's pronounced it wrong, the Hole might dump him somewhere at random, or inside a mountain or something awful like that!' said Dirk.

220

'Well...' said Sooz, rubbing her chin.

'Come on, what did he say, exactly?' said Dirk.

Sooz sighed. 'He said...he said, "The Goblin Warrens". I'm sorry, Dirk!'

Dirk's face fell. Betrayed? By a Goblin? And he'd treated him so well, more like a friend than a minion, feeding him corned beef and custard and stuff. Hah, that's what you got for being a softie!

'Oooo, that little...' said Dirk, his hands clawing up in anger.

'Terrible cowards, Goblins,' said Rufino. 'Always were – not like Orcs.'

'So, what – he just went home, is that it?' said Chris.

'Yes, indeed,' said Dirk, a little calmer now. 'Home to the Goblin Warrens. I should have known after the last time.'

'Doesn't really matter, though – we still have Gargon and Rufino and the Ring,' said Sooz.

'By the Dark Gods, of course, the Ring!' said Dirk, holding up his hand and gazing at the great Ring of Power.

It was glowing, the runes coruscating with crimson fire, a strange, dark light emanating from it, shrouding Dirk in its magic. Dirk turned to look at his shadow – it was huge, goat-legged and horned, just like his Dark Lord form, before the Essence of Evil was sucked out of him, cursing him into the body of a puny human boy.

Dirk admired the shadow, and cackled to himself. 'Anyway, we'll deal with Skinrash later!' he said.

'You won't...you know, be too harsh or kill him or anything, will you?' said Sooz, exchanging a nervous glance with Chris. The last time they were in the Darklands with Dirk and the Ring, things hadn't turned out so well.[1]

'No, no, of course not! I'm a Dark Lord, sure, but the boy, not the beast. I'll just put him on latrine duty or something,' said Dirk.

They were standing in a bleached-bone cleft of mountain rock. On three sides, the mountain rose up, pale and rocky, to a bright blue sky. Wisps of volcanic smoke came from the peaks.

'Welcome to the High Sierra of the Ash Mountains,' said Dirk. 'Down that ridge a way, you'll find pleasanter climes, where the Highland

1. Read *Dark Lord: A Fiend in Need* to find out what happened last time.

Orcs grow crops on their terraces, raise mountain goats, and live in their caves and hill forts, raiding down into the Borderlands from time to time. But up here, no one comes.'

'I suppose that's the entrance, right?' said Rufino, pointing to a yawning black opening in the mountainside nearby.

'Yes, the Caverns of Grief, the Lair of the Black Hag,' said Dirk portentously, gesturing at the yawning maw with his ring hand. The Ring trailed wisps of darkness as it moved.

Everyone gazed at the Cavern's mouth with trepidation, until Chris broke the spell.

'Well, no point in hanging about,' he said, setting off towards it.

He was no coward, you had to give him that, thought Dirk to himself.

They trudged over, their feet throwing up little puffs of pale ash. Soon they arrived at the Cavern's entrance. They stood for a moment, staring at the dark opening, the dragon's maw, the lion's mouth. Did they really have to go in?

# The Lady Grieves – But For Whom?

Into the unknown they stepped.

They expected some kind of relief from the dry heat, but although it was cooler, it was still dry and parched in the dark cave.

The band of intrepid adventurers paused to get their bearings. Dirk held up his ring hand – from it pulsed a shadowy grey light. It did not dispel the dark like regular light, rather it replaced the dark with something that was...well, less dark.

They were in a vast cavern of crumbling rock. Underfoot, bones and ash crunched – animal bones mostly, by the look of them. At least they weren't human bones, which was a small comfort to Sooz and Chris. Directly overhead, the roof was so far away it was shrouded in shadow. But it sloped down ahead to meet with the walls that slanted in at the sides, leading to a large, square-topped archway.

All was quiet.

'Come on,' whispered Dirk. He didn't want to give their position away, but also the caverns were filled with a sinister ambience, as of the grave. It made everyone feel that to make too much noise was to break some kind of rule.

They walked on in silence, up to the big portal. Two great uprights and a lintel of pale white stone formed the squared-off arch. The bone-white stone radiated in the grey light of the Ring with a kind of sickly pallor. Runes were carved into the pillars.

Dirk looked at them closely. 'Ah, as I thought,' he whispered. 'Shadowglyphs of the Black Tongue!'

'What does it say?' said Chris.

'Hah, you have hit the nail on the bed there, Christopher,' said Dirk, reaching out to the Runes with his hand.

'Head, nail on the *head*,' said Sooz, without thinking.

Chris giggled, though not for long. The oppressive gloom crushed all laughter and joy in a heartbeat.

Dirk paused, hand outstretched. He blinked for a moment. 'Right, on the head, of course,' he whispered.

'You cannot read these Runes, Christopher, you see,' whispered Rufino. 'You can only hear them.'

'And only those who are truly of the Dark can make the Shadowglyphs speak,' said Dirk quietly. He ran his fingers over the Runes. As he did so, each Shadowglyph made a sound, the sounds coming together as words and sentences.

A voice murmured into their ears, like waves gently lapping at a shore of corpses.

'Herein Lies the Land from which No One Returns.'

'I suppose we're just going to ignore this, and go in, right?' said Chris.

'I suppose – hah, imagine what Mum would say!' said Sooz.

'What do you mean?' whispered Dirk, curiously.

'Well you know... Umm... "Hi, Mum, I'm just going out." "Where are you going, dear?" "Just popping to the Land from which No One Returns, Mum." "Oh all right then, dear, see you later!"'

'Or not,' added Chris with a grin.

'Well, do not fear, little ones. Be of stout heart, and we shall prevail!' said Rufino in a low voice.

'Pah, typical Paladin optimism – it'll be my Ring

and the mighty Gargon that'll do the prevailing!' said Dirk under his breath. 'Come on then, let's go.'

With that he stepped through the portal, the others following close behind. They walked into a huge, vaulted hallway, carved from the rock long, long ago. Massive statues of robed skeletons lined the walls. Chipped and crumbling, the decaying statues rose up and bent over, holding up the ceiling on their hunched shoulders, skeletal arms outstretched across the roof like a web of bony vines.

'What is this place?' said Rufino, staring up in awe at the vastness of it.

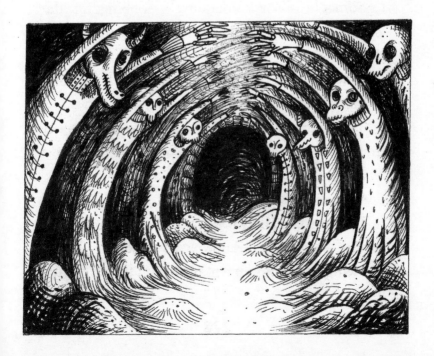

'I don't know,' said Dirk. 'It is ancient beyond reckoning, even for one such as I.'

They moved through the gloom slowly.

Suddenly, a sound disturbed the darkness.

'What was that?' hissed Sooz. They strained their ears. Up ahead, a faint sound – there, again!

They advanced. The vaulted ceiling gave way to raw crumbling rock, the hallway narrowing fast, filled with fallen boulders, jumbled pillars and cracked statues where it had all collapsed in. The sound grew louder...small cries in the distance.

As of someone crying.

Someone – or something – sobbing, in the shadows. It unnerved them all, the sound of weeping in the dark.

'It is the Lady Grieve,' whispered Dirk. 'She mourns for her victims.'

They came to a halt. Up ahead, a pile of fallen rock had left only a small opening. There was no way Gargon could get through. Rufino, at a pinch, by wriggling. Gargon never.

Dirk put a hand up to his face in thought. He looked Gargon up and down. 'Maybe if we removed his wings...' he muttered to himself.

Gargon stared back at him in horror.

'We can't do that!' hissed Sooz.

'No, no, don't think it would work anyway,' Dirk mumbled. He turned to examine the gap in the jumbled rock.

'What if you used the Ring to blast a way through?' said Rufino quietly.

'I was thinking about that,' murmured Dirk. 'But, looking around...' Everywhere were piles of loose rock and crumbled stone. 'I'd be risking bringing the whole mountain down on top of us!'

As if to underline his words, a stream of dust and pebbles slooshed down one side of the tunnel, trickling to a stop at Gargon's great, gnarled feet.

'It could block the way completely. Bury us even. No, I think we'll just have to go on without Gargon,' said Dirk.

'Without old Gargie? But he's our best fighter!' said Sooz.

Dirk shrugged. 'No choice,' he said.

'Gargon sorry, my lady. Gargon just too big. And Gargon want to keep his wings.'

Rufino shook his head. 'Can't think of a way round it, I'm afraid. Gargon will have to stay.'

'Me stay here, wait for you to come back?' said Gargon.

'No, no point, my Dread Lieutenant. When we've got what we want, we'll use the crystal to go straight back to Earth. Nope, you head off, back to the Iron Tower. Rest up a bit, say hello to Agrash. When we get back, I'll send Dave with a message, let you know we're OK.'

'And if no message from Dave?' said Gargon.

'Then you'll know we died here,' said Dirk.

'Well, at least we know we won't die unmourned,' said Rufino.

'Quite so,' said Dirk. 'The Black Hag will give us a good funeral, that's for sure!'

'Well, goodbye then old Gargie,' said Sooz. 'Hopefully see you later!'

'Farewell, my Dark Lady,' said the great beast, 'Gargon see you soon.'

'See if you can get Agrash to make you a guitar. You gotta keep practising – when this is over, we'll do a gig in the Darklands or something.'

'Cool, my Queen, Gargon love to play!'

'All right, all right, enough of that. Come on, we're on a quest here, not a musicians' night out!'

said Dirk with irritation. Although it was really the fact that Gargon obviously preferred Sooz to him that annoyed him. Anyway, whatever.

He stepped into the dark opening, beckoning the others to follow.

Sooz held Gargon's hand for a moment, before turning away. Gargon watched them disappear into the gloom, his fiendish red eyes filling with unshed tears.

Beyond the narrow gate was a dusty tunnel. Here, the sound of sobbing filled the air all around them. The hot and dusty air. Each of them was parched and thirsty, each of them envying Gargon, each wishing it was all over, so that they could go home for a nice meal and a long, cold drink of lemonade.

They trudged on. The tunnel narrowed. And narrowed. Until they had to crouch down. And down.

Now they had to crawl.

The darkness closed in around them like a black, suffocating blanket. The sound of quiet sobbing filled their ears. Eventually, the way opened into a small chamber, a little egg of space inside the heart of the mountain.

Ahead lay a small opening from which echoed the sobs of the Lady Grieve. The four of them stared at it, worried looks on their grey-lit faces.

It was obvious Rufino would never get through. And he had no wings to cut off...

Dirk groaned in frustration. 'Ten thousand curses on the heads of fluffy little bunny rabbits!' he shouted in anger. His words echoed around the tunnels and back at them like a tannoy.

'...fluffy little bunny rabbits...'

'...fluffy little bunny rabbits...'

'...fluffy little bunny rabbits...'

Abruptly, the sobbing stopped.

Dirk put a hand up to his mouth. 'Sorry,' he hissed through his fingers.

'She knows we're here,' said Sooz.

'Advantage of surprise lost,' said Chris.

'And I can't come with you,' said Rufino.

Dirk put his face in his hands.

'Perhaps we should give it up, try another strategy for dealing with Hasdruban,' said Rufino.

They stood in silence for a moment, thinking.

'But what?' said Dirk. 'What else is there? We will never get another chance to come back here, and if we go back to Earth, eventually Hasdruban will succeed.'

'And kill you,' said Chris.

'Right,' said Sooz. 'We have no choice, we'll have to go on alone, the three of us.'

'You are brave indeed!' said Rufino. 'I shall wait here for your return.'

'No, no – same applies to you as to Gargon. We'll either die here or go straight home to Earth.'

Rufino hesitated for a moment. Then he sighed. 'You are right, there is nothing for it.'

'Go and find Gargon. Go home to the Iron Tower, we'll be in touch!'

'Yeah,' said Sooz, 'and look after my town – you know, Soozville.'

'I will my Lady, farewell, and good luck. I will see you soon, I'm sure!' He shook each of them by the hand, and then saluted formally, as was the way with Paladins. He was turning to go when Sooz rushed forward and gave him a hug.

'Thank you, Rufino, for being my friend,' she said.

Rufino smiled down at her. 'It has been my honour to serve you,' he replied.

Dirk raised his eyes. 'Oh please, come on!' he said.

'Goodbye Rufey,' said Sooz, before turning away and glaring at Dirk.

'What?' said Dirk.

'Let's just get on with it, shall we?' said Chris.

# The Lair of the Black Hag

The three children found themselves in a large open space, a natural cave in the heart of the mountain. Far off to the side, pools of red hot lava bubbled and belched sedately, filling the cavern with a reddish glow but also with an oppressive heat worse even than what they had experienced so far. Ancient and massive stalactites and stalagmites created a panorama of jagged chaos. Threads of quartz ran through the rock, glittering with ruby radiance.

It would have been beautiful, if it was not also the Lair of the Black Hag.

Up ahead, past the forest of dripstone trees, they could see what looked like a door, set in the far wall of the cavern.

They advanced towards it, a terrible thirst

beginning to build up inside them. Dirk led the way, ring finger pointing ahead, ready to release the Blast of Ravening Flame at a moment's notice. In the lava glow, the Runes writhed with a fiery intensity like never before.

Suddenly, a ragged figure stepped out from behind a squat stalagmite. The Black Hag! She stood there, arms at her side, talons outspread, a tattered black-lace assassin from your worst nightmare.

'Oh myyy,' she rasped in a voice as dry as bone, 'How nice of you to come and visit, my pretties, how nice. I shall have the most delightful funeral party this afternoon, oh yes!'

The Black Hag stepped forward.

Dirk pointed a finger. 'Stay right there, Lady Grieve, for though I am trapped in the body of a puny human, I am still the Dark Lord, and I wield the Great Ring!' With that he unleashed a Blast of Ravening Flame with a thunderous crack. A bolt of flame leaped forward, and struck the squat stalagmite next to the Black Hag.

The stalagmite shattered into tiny pieces, showering the Hag in jagged shards. She jumped back in shock, and then fell to her knees, next to another chunky stalagmite.

'My Lord,' shrieked the Hag. 'Stay your dread hand, I beg you, I did not know!' she shrieked, clasping her hands pleadingly, the talons clicking together to form a briar of envenomed iron.

Chris folded his arms, relieved at how well it seemed to be going whilst Sooz put her arms on her hips. 'Typical bully!' she muttered.

Dirk grinned.

'Too easy, if you ask me,' said Chris.

'*Bah*, nonsense, she just sees me for what I really am!' said Dirk dismissively. 'Don't you, my Lady? Finally, you know your place,' he said, drawing himself up to his full height, enhanced by the power of the Ring, which also added a certain dark majesty to his imperious tones.

The Black Hag bowed her head in submission. Dirk glanced at Chris triumphantly. He turned back to the kneeling Hag.

'I will spare you, despite your treachery, but on one condition!' said Dirk.

'Name it, your Dark Majesty!' said the Black Hag, bowing her head.

'I need a tear or two, that is all,' said Dirk.

The Lady Grieve looked up, put a hand out to rest on the stalagmite beside her, opened the other iron-nailed hand in a gesture of acquiescence.

'I have cried many tears of grief,' she said.

Suddenly, she pushed at the stalagmite – a secret door clicked open!

'And I shall cry some more over your dead bodies!' she shrieked as she disappeared into the interior of the stalagmite before Dirk could do a thing.

Gathering his wits, Dirk leaped forward but only in time to hear the secret door clicking shut. Desperately he felt around, pushing and pulling and shoving, but nothing moved.

'Told you!' said Chris.

Dirk growled under his breath, stepped back, and angrily blasted the stalagmite with the Ring. It blew up with a roar, scattering dust and crystal everywhere. But no sign of the Black Hag.

'Whoa!' said Sooz, 'Careful, Dirk, what if she'd been still inside and you'd killed her! We need her alive.'

Dirk made a face. 'You're right, I know. I just lost it there for a moment.'

'Anyway, where'd she go?' said Chris.

'I don't know. Secret passageway, I guess,' said Sooz.

'Well... Let us go on, head for the door. I bet that's her Inner Sanctum, perhaps we can find some tears in there,' said Dirk.

The three drew together, Dirk in front, Ring at the ready, and they set off for the door, threading their way through the limestone forest.

A minute passed. They were drawing nearer. Another minute.

A sudden loud click...and out of a nearby stalagmite leaped the Black Hag! With a cry of, 'A contract's a contract!' she raked a taloned hand down Dirk's arm before anyone could say or do anything. He gasped in pain, turned, ring at the ready, but the Hag had jumped back behind the secret door.

Dirk fell to his knees, burning agony racing up his arm. He just had enough strength to blast the stalagmite to pieces with his Ring, but then he fell back to the ground, lying there, barely able to move.

In the distance, a witchy cackling echoed around the caverns.

'Dirk, no!' yelled Sooz, as she ran to his side.

Chris looked on, his face pale and shocked.

A thin lattice of black lines began to form under Dirk's skin. Beads of sweat sprang up on his brow.

'Paralysis...setting in...quick...need antidote!' Dirk ground out through gritted teeth, his face rigid with agony.

Hurriedly, Sooz fumbled in her pocket, drew out the little bottle of antidote Dirk had given her, and poured it down his throat.

Dirk began to gasp for breath, taking in long rattling gulps of air... Sooz took him by the hand. 'No, don't die, Dirk, please don't die!' she said, her eyes filling with tears. Dirk looked up at her. He squeezed her hand. He could not speak.

But then the pain began to ease. He could breathe again. The filigree of black that laced his skin began to fade. Sooz put a hand to his forehead.

'You're going to be all right,' she said, 'It's working!'

'Thank you, Sooz,' said Dirk.

Sooz patted his hand. 'I think maybe we should give up on this, time to go home, don't you think?' she said.

Dirk sat up, coughing. 'That's better...and no, we can't go back. I will not let that evil Hag defeat us!'

he said defiantly. 'I still have the Ring, have I not?'

'But it's so dangerous,' said Chris. 'I mean, what if it's me next, or worse, Sooz!'

'*Bah*, I never give up!' said Dirk.

Chris shook his head. 'This is bonkers – we're just kids, Dirk!'

Dirk got to his feet. 'Well, I shall never give up, you can if you want.'

'Chris is right, Dirk, you've got to see reason here! We can try something else to defeat Hasdruban when we get back – you're a genius, Dirk, you can come up with something, right?' said Sooz.

'I admire your flattery technique, my dear little Goth, but really, we must go on. I mean, this is our best chance, if we go back without the tear...well, Hasdruban will get me in the end, don't you see? He's the headmaster, he's holding most of the cards!'

Chris stood there, arms folded. 'That's a fair point,' he said.

Sooz frowned. Then she stood up, with her back to the sitting Dirk, and nodded at Chris's satchel.

Chris looked at her. He raised a quizzical eyebrow. She nodded urgently, at the satchel.

'Use the crystal,' she whispered. 'Now!'

Dirk, oblivious, looked around. 'These stalagmites are probably riddled with secret passages. Maybe if I start blasting all the ones in the way, we could clear a safe path,' he mused. 'If only I wasn't so thirsty!'

Chris put a hand to his chin, thinking. Then he reached into his satchel, but instead of getting the Anathema Crystal he pulled out the flask, inscribed with 'The Dark Lord', the flask he was going to give as a gift to Dirk.

Chris paused for a moment, unsure. Then he seemed to make up his mind, and he said, 'Here you are, Dirk – I got you this as a present!'

'By the Nine Hells, Chris, thank you!' said Dirk, putting out his hand to Sooz, and nodding up at her so that she'd pass him the flask.

Sooz reached over, took the flask, and began to pass it over to Dirk.

'Have a drink, it'll quench your thirst for sure,' said Chris.

Sooz paused. 'Let's have a swig then,' she said, 'I'm dying of thirst too!' She flipped up the lid, and put the flask to her mouth.

'NOOOOOOOOO!' yelled Chris at the top of his voice. But it was too late, Sooz had taken a sip.

Sooz's eyes widened at Chris's cry – she was about to yank the flask away from her lips but then she tasted whatever it was that was in the flask. And she couldn't help herself. It tasted like...liberation. Freedom. No more rules, no more behaving yourself. Just Sooz, doing whatever Sooz wanted. She began to gulp it down, all of it, gulp after gulp.

'What? What is it?' Dirk said, confusion written all over his face, as he heaved himself to his feet.

Chris looked over at Dirk, his face full of fear and horror at what he'd done. He stepped back... 'Essence of Evil, Dirk,' he said. 'Essence of Evil!'

# Sooz, the Vampire Queen

Sooz let the flask fall from her nerveless fingers to clatter on the stony cavern floor. Her eyes rolled up, showing only the whites. Her head began to shake and shiver, until her features started to blur.

Chris put a hand up to his face. 'No, no, no,' he kept saying. Dirk stepped back, a mixture of horror and fascination on his face.

Sooz's arms were jerking about, crooked and broken-looking. Her legs began to lengthen. She began to grow...

Suddenly, she was engulfed in a cloud of black smoke that seemed to come out of nowhere. It roiled and bubbled, shot through with crimson streaks before seeming to suddenly disappear *into* her.

Leaving a new Sooz...

She stood tall, nearly as tall as Gargon. Her old clothes had morphed and been re-stitched into a full black bodysuit under a massive cloak of blood red velvet with a bat-wing collar of glossy black. She still wore her chunky Goth boots but somehow the Essence of Evil had made them bigger than ever.

She stared down at Chris and Dirk, her skin pale as ivory, her nails black and glossy, her hair long and black with streaks of white, a tiara of jagged, ruby-studded silver on her head. Her eyes were red. Completely red, even the whites. Two white fangs protruded over her crimson lips...

Dirk's jaw dropped. 'Sooz, the Vampire Queen!' he said in awed tones.

Chris reached for his satchel.

'Don't you dare use that crystal, boy!' said Sooz in rich tones like chocolate. Chocolate and death, that is.

She stepped closer to Chris, who had frozen in place, his face a mask of fear.

Sooz reached a hand out towards him, as if she were going to seize him up and drink his blood. But then she paused.

'Christopher,' she said. 'Put the satchel down, there's a good boy. Don't make me...eat you.'

Chris dropped the satchel, terrified. Sooz turned

to Dirk. He was staring at her.

'You are awesome, Sooz, awesome!' he said.

Sooz smiled, revealing perfect white teeth and fangs.

'Of course you'd become a Vampire, what else?' said Dirk.

Sooz nodded. 'It is rather cool,' she said.

'OK, my sweet little Vampire,' said Dirk. 'You know what happened with me last time I was the Dark Lord – it'll happen to you too. I can't allow you to harm Chris. Or me, for that matter. I think all in all it is best that you let Chris use the crystal, we all return home, and you will be changed back into the real, nice, kind Sooz that we all love.'

With that, he raised his Ring and pointed it at Sooz.

Sooz raised an eyebrow. And then leaned forward, her face transformed into angry malice.

'You would never dare! Blast me with the Ring then, go on, do it, little boy!' she hissed.

Dirk blinked up at her. She was right, he couldn't... not to Sooz. And she was magnificent as a Vampire, magnificent!

'You see, Dirk, I know you now, I know what it all means! Without this power, this greatness, this Essence of Wonder, we are weak! Wretched and pitiful,

246

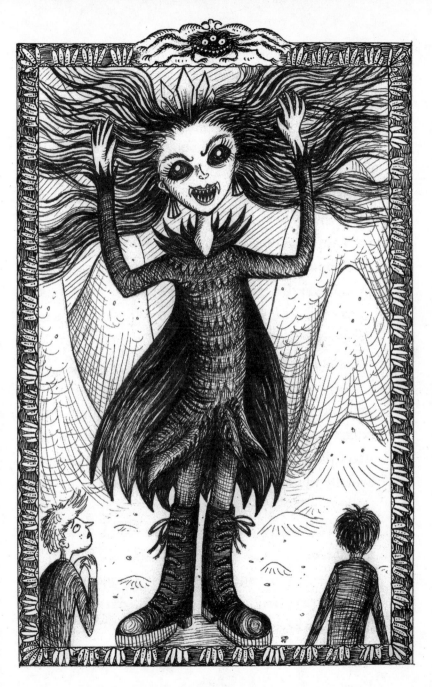

*Susan Black from Sussex*

hobbled by conscience and do-gooding foolishness!'

Dirk shook his head, 'No, no, that's not you talking, it's...'

'Silence, child!' shrieked Sooz into his face. 'Now, give me the Ring. Immediately!'

Dirk put his hand behind his back and stepped away.

'Never,' he said.

'Don't do this, Sooz,' said Chris.

Sooz waved a pale hand dismissively.

'Give me the Ring, Dirk, or use it. Your choice,' she said silkily.

'I...I can't,' said Dirk.

Suddenly, with an inarticulate cry of rage, Sooz stepped forward and grabbed Dirk roughly. She pulled his arm up to her face with the irresistible strength of the vampire, grabbed the Ring and brutally yanked it off his finger, tearing the skin.

Dirk gasped in pain.

Sooz stared at the small trickle of blood on Dirk's finger, her face full of Vampire madness.

But then she seemed to pull herself together. She stepped back, shaking her head as if to clear it. Dirk sank to his knees, grimacing in pain.

'I'm...sorry, Dirk,' said Sooz, 'I just lost control!' She stepped forward as if to comfort him, but Chris put a hand out.

'Back, Vampire!' he said. 'Before you do something worse!'

A red tear appeared at the corner of her eye. 'I didn't mean... I don't know what came over me, it was... I'm sorry!'

The tear trickled down one cheek, leaving a tiny river of blood down the side of her face. But then Sooz noticed the Great Ring of Power in her hand, and her guilt was forgotten.

'Well, it's only a scratch,' she said, 'I'm sure you'll get over it!'

Sooz put the Ring on. Immediately she took on an aura of even greater infernal magnificence, radiating power and strength. But also evil. A terrible and hungry evil.

'This is brill!' she said. 'With this Ring I shall be the greatest of all the Queens of the Darklands. Goodbye Moon Queen, hello Queen of Vampires!'

The Ring glowed and coruscated with energy as if it were pleased to be on her hand.

'Good to have you back again,' said Sooz to the

Ring. 'But this time...well...we shall see. I'm going to have so much fun!'

The Vampire Queen turned, her crimson robe swirling, her pale face and ruby lips lit up with the reddish glow of hot lava. At her feet, two children huddled, staring up at her fearfully.

Sooz looked down at them and smiled. 'My little pets...or perhaps sweet little snacks?'

But then she frowned. 'Maybe it is best you two return to Earth before I do something I will regret... I will rule here now on my own.'

'What about the tear?' said Dirk.

'Ah yes, of course,' said Sooz. 'Hmm, I think I can sort that out for you!'

'What do you mean?' said Chris.

'I'll find the Black Hag, force her to give up a tear or die, give it you. Simples!' said the Vampire Queen. 'I mean – the Black Hag vs Sooz the Vampire Queen with the Great Ring? Who's gonna win?'

'Right,' said Dirk.

'Back in a jiffy,' said Sooz. She turned away in a crimson swirl, heading towards the door at the far end of the cavern. Dirk and Chris watched her go. She suddenly shot forward with blinding, inhuman speed, leaving a trail of wispy darkness in the air behind her.

When she was out of earshot, Dirk rounded on Chris.

'What the Nine Hells were you doing? You tried to make me drink the Essence! I mean, why, for goodness sake, why?'

Chris put his head in his hands. 'I'm sorry, Dirk. I... I wanted you to drink it, I admit it.'

'But why – you're my...my brother! Why'd you do that to me, you knew I didn't want to be that kind of Dark Lord any more!'

Chris stared at him. 'Well... I wanted...partly it was a last-ditch thing. You know, so that you'd be the Dark Lord, the real thing. You'd be able to beat the Black Hag easily.'

'Ah, I see! And then...you'd use the crystal, get us all back? I'd turn back into me? Not a bad plan, actually. Risky, though, you know what I'd be like as the Dark Lord and I'd have known you had a crystal!' said Dirk.

Chris stared at the floor. Almost imperceptibly he shook his head.

Dirk raised a puzzled eyebrow. 'What?' said Dirk.

'What then?'

'I was going to use the crystal, but just for me and Sooz...'

Dirk gasped. 'And leave me here in the Darklands!'

'Yes,' said Chris. 'In your rightful place, as the ruler, where you belong. Leaving me and Sooz as we used to be, back home, just ordinary people, together. Without you telling me what to do, making me feel small, using me!'

Dirk stared in open-mouthed amazement. 'I can't believe it!' was all he could say.

'What do you expect! You treat me like your servant. You think I'm worthless,' said Chris.

'No, no, not worthless, just...'

'Shut up and listen for once! You come to our home – my home – and cause trouble. You hid a Goblin in the cupboard. A Goblin! You upset my mum and my dad – ruined my mum's contact lenses, made her see weird stuff, and you made her faint! You got me blamed for stealing a cake. You put a Goblin axe in the headmaster's study – nearly got us all arrested. And that's just in the past few days! Then there's the psycho nanny who came into the house because of you and cast a spell on my parents.

You burned down the cricket pavilion, we nearly got expelled. That White Beast thing nearly ripped me up, and then I was almost sacrificed on an altar by Skirrits, *because of you*. And I had to wear pink underpants with hearts on, not to mention that stinking stuff they covered me in. And then after that you cut my face, leaving a scar for ever, and locked me in a dungeon. And now, I'm in a cave with a poisonous Hag and my best friend is a Vampire!'

Dirk put a hand up to his chin. 'Well, when you put it like that...' he said.

# Love and Kisses, Darklands Style

Suddenly there was a crash like thunder from up ahead.

'The Ring!' said Dirk.

There was a loud shriek, and another crash. What was going on? Was Sooz all right?

And then laughter. Not the witchy cackling of the Hag, but a rich bell-like laugh, resonant with evil.

'Heh, heh, heh!' it went, echoing around the Caverns.

'Sooz's version of 'Mwah, hah, hah', I think,' said Chris.

'Sounds like it,' said Dirk. He turned to Chris suddenly. 'You're right, Chris. I haven't treated you well. And I have caused you a lot of grief and suffering. I'm sorry.'

Chris looked at him. He sighed a heavy sigh. 'It's

OK, Dirk, I know you didn't mean to do all that. It's just...what you do, I guess.'

'So I'm forgiven then?' said Dirk.

'Yeah, yeah, and I'm sorry I pulled the trick with the...hold on a minute!' said a surprised Chris. 'You just apologised. Dark Lords never apologise!'

Dirk looked away. '*Bah*, I'm not the Dark Lord I once was, I suppose. And anyway, you have to say sorry to your friends sometimes, right? Especially your brother!'

Chris smiled at him. It felt good to hear Dirk say those words.

'Yeah, bro,' he said, putting a hand on Dirk's shoulder. 'Anyway, how's the finger?'

'Hurts a bit, but Sooz is right. It's only a scratch.'

Chris raised an eyebrow. 'You evil overlord types are weird,' he said.

'Here she comes,' said Dirk, nodding towards the far end of the Cavern. Striding towards them came the Vampire Queen, wreathed in crimson, every now and then flickering forwards like a flashing blade.

'Give me the crystal!' said Dirk. 'She thinks you've got it, but maybe I can get close enough to use it.'

Chris nodded, and handed it over. But then he said, 'What if she keeps me away or something. What if I don't get caught in the crystal? I'll be stuck here with the Hag!'

'Good point,' said Dirk. 'If that happens, when the time comes I'll shout, "NOW!" When you hear that, run in as fast as you can. I'll make sure the crystal gets all of us.'

Sooz came up, with a fanged grin on her face. In one hand she held a bottle, small but stout, and some torn up tattered black lace in the other. She stood some distance away, just out of crystal range.

She held up the bottle.

'Here's the tear, my dear!' she said.

'Is the Hag dead?' said Dirk.

'Oh no, she's far too pretty to kill. Not to mention useful!' said Sooz. 'No, we came to...an agreement.'

'So, can I have the tear,' said Dirk, taking a step forward.

'Stay where you are!' barked the Vampire Queen. 'I know you've got that crystal, and you'll be planning to use it, trying to "save me from myself" or some such meddling nonsense!'

'Chris has the crystal,' said Dirk.

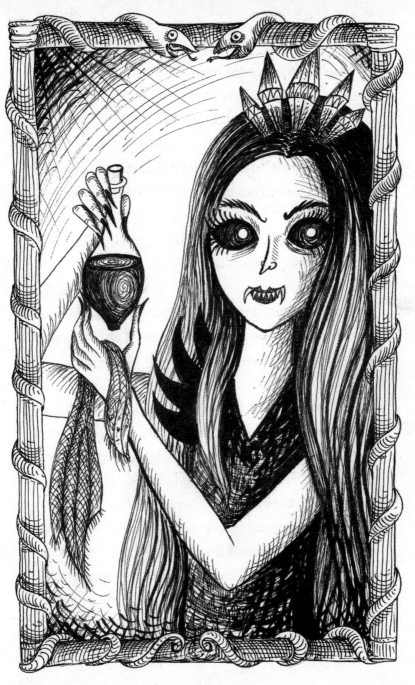

*Tears before bedtime*

'Sue me for not taking your word on that, little Dirkikins!' said Sooz.

'Don't call me that!' said Dirk.

Sooz laughed. 'In fact, step away from each other. Go on, Chris, at least ten feet apart, behind Dirk as far as you can get from me. No crystal trickery here!'

Dirk nodded at Chris. They moved apart. Not quite ten feet, but almost.

'There you are, Dirkikins. I got several tears, more than enough, I would think,' said Sooz, as she tossed over the bottle. It clattered at Dirk's feet. Dirk reached down and picked it up.

'Now,' continued Sooz, 'go and join Chris, use the crystal and get out of here before I change my mind, take you back to the Iron Tower and lock you in the Dungeons of Doom, just like you did to me.'

Dirk put his hands on his hips. 'All very well, but how are you going to get out of here? You're as big as Rufino now!' he said.

'Oh please, don't you think I've thought of that? The Black Hag – in return for her life – showed me a different way out. The whole mountain

258

is riddled with secret passages.'

'And you trusted her?' said Dirk.

'Oh yes – she knows perfectly well that if she's lying I could drain her dry in a second – in this form, I'm much, much faster than she is, and Vampires are immune to poison,' said Sooz.

Dirk looked at her. Nobody spoke.

After a few moments, Sooz said, 'Face it, Dirk, you have to go home, and I'll stay here. Hey, look on the bright side! You've got a chance with the tears of the Lady Grieve. If you can't pull it off, I'll be raising an army of Orcs and Goblins, anyway, and invading the Commonwealth. Hasdruban will have to come back to defend his lands. Then I'll defeat him and drink his blood, probably.'

Dirk and Chris exchanged glances, their faces pale. It was really awful to hear Sooz speak like this.

'What about Rufino?' said Dirk.

Sooz frowned. 'Rufino...' she muttered.

'You can't kill him!' said Chris.

'No, no, I can't do that. No, I'll probably exile him or something,' said Sooz.

Chris and Dirk stared up at the Vampire Queen.

'So this is it?' said Chris. 'After all we've been

through, we're just going to split up?'

'Yup. It's better this way. You know what happened with Dirk when he was the Dark Lord? Same thing's going to happen to me, it's inevitable.'

'But, but...' said Chris.

'Don't worry about me! I've always wanted to be a Vampire, haven't I?' said Sooz.

'Yeah, but not a proper one, not like this...' said Chris.

Sooz shrugged, the bat wing collars of her Vampire cloak rising and falling.

'Well, so be it, come on over, Chris, use the crystal on us both,' Dirk said, beckoning to Chris.

Chris stood there confused. Dirk had the crystal...

'Come on, you idiot, we haven't got all day, we might as well head back – no point wasting time with Sooz any more, right?'

Chris took an uncertain step forward, not sure what Dirk's plan was.

'Stay where you are, Chris, Dirk should be going to you!' said Sooz, her voice commanding him in an almost hypnotic way.

Chris froze, as if he'd been enchanted. But now he understood. Dirk had tricked Sooz into thinking

Chris had the crystal. Clever...

Meanwhile, Sooz put her hands on her hips, and stamped a heavily booted foot into the cavern floor, raising up a small cloud of dust.

'And anyway, what do you mean, "wasting time with Sooz"! Is that what you really think, Dirk, you nasty little...boy!' she said getting more and more angry.

'Well, you want to be Vampire Queen, fine. No skin off my nose, won't kiss you or miss you,' he said.

Sooz's eyes widened with rage. 'You won't...oooh, you...' She stepped a little closer, her hands balled into fists, her eyes glowing with rage. 'You won't miss me when you're dead either!'

'You wouldn't kill me,' said Dirk. 'After all, you love me too much, don't you?'

'What!' said Sooz, stepping even closer. 'Why would I love...' But then her voice faltered, different emotions warring for control – good and evil, love and...well, general Vampire stuff.

Dirk looked up at her. 'Actually, I *would* miss you,' he said, his eyes filling up with water. 'You see, Sooz, I love you.'

Sooz's jaw dropped and then she seemed to light up. All right, she lit up with a reddish, pale, ghostly vampiric glow, but still, it was light. She beamed a great, fanged smile.

'Oh, Dirk,' she said, stepping up to him, 'I love you too!'

'NOW, Chris, now!' said Dirk, as he drew out the crystal, ready to throw it at their feet.

Chris, whose heart had just been pierced by a dagger of jealousy at the exchange of love vows between Dirk and Sooz, was a little slow off the mark. Nevertheless, he dived forward, but Dirk was still forced to delay hurling the crystal to the floor.

And that gave Sooz time to act. She was fast, Vampire fast. 'You tricked me!' she yelled, a high-pitched Vampire shriek. She grabbed his wrist and ripped the crystal right out of his hand. Holding the crystal in one hand, she grabbed Dirk with the other and stuck her face in his.

'I'm going to kill you!' she hissed, baring her fangs and spraying Dirk's face with Vampire saliva.

Dirk spoke fast and desperately. 'I did it for you! Because I love you, because I wanted to save you!'

Sooz blinked at him for a moment, half convinced.

Dirk wiped the saliva off his face and then narrowed his eyes – he'd just had an idea.

Suddenly he leaned forward and kissed Sooz. Her eyes widened in surprise.

Sooz began to struggle, trying to break free from the kiss. Something strange began to happen. Sooz, the Vampire Queen, stronger, faster, deadlier than Dirk, couldn't break free. Some force was holding her in place, and it wasn't Dirk.

She began to shrink and dwindle, her skin colour becoming more healthy and human. At the same time, Dirk began to grow, his body changing into his Dark Lord form, huge horns sprouting from his head, his legs turning into great goat-hoofed tree trunks, black talons sprouting from his hands, skeletal bone bursting out all over his face.

The Essence of Evil was returning to its rightful home, the body of the Dark Lord. It didn't really belong inside a thirteen-year-old schoolgirl from Sussex, even if she did make for a rather cool Vampire, had the Great Ring of Power, and once ruled over the Darklands as the Moon Queen. It belonged inside the Dark Lord, it *was* the Dark Lord.

Sooz was Sooz again, and she sat down suddenly, weak, wretched and exhausted. Chris ran over, knelt down beside her and put a hand around her shoulder. Dirk, meanwhile, stood up to his full Dark Lord height, leaned back his head and shouted.

'I'M BACK! MWAH, HAH, HAH!' The great laugh of the Dark Lord echoed around the cavern like thunder.

Sooz looked down at her hand. In it she held an Anathema Crystal. She looked at Chris, who nodded back at her. She raised her hand...

'No, wait!' said Dirk. 'I've changed my mind, I want to be a Dark Lord after all!'

Sooz threw the crystal to the floor. It shattered into pieces, throwing up a cloud of iridescent diamond dust, engulfing all three of them. The Dark Lord stared down in horror.

'AIEEE, I've outwitted myself!' he howled as they all began to fall....

# 'Girlfriend' Trouble

Dirk was sitting in his room, concentrating on the task at hand. He had a bag of wine gums, and he was injecting the black tears of the Lady Grieve into each one. There was a knock on the door.

Dirk frowned in irritation and muttered to himself, 'Can't these accursed humans leave me alone, even for a minute?' Then he sighed, and said loudly, 'Who is it?'

'It's me, Sooz!' said a voice. Then she opened the door and walked in.

'We need to talk,' she said. She seemed rather nervous.

Dirk turned to face her. 'What about? Everything's good, isn't it?' he said.

'About...you know, what happened,' said Sooz, twisting a finger into her dyed black hair.

'What?' said Dirk.

'You know...in that cave,' said Sooz.

'Yeah, you turned into a Vampire, it was "well cold", as they say!'

'Well cool! And no, not that bit – the other...the other bit!' said Sooz.

Dirk frowned. 'You sound like Chris. What are you on about?'

'You know! The kiss, you moron! THE KISS!' she said, stamping her foot.

'Oh, that!' said Dirk. 'Um, yeah, whatever,' he added, shrugging.

Sooz folded her arms and glared at Dirk. 'Whatever? That's all you've got to say about it? WHATEVER! Right, well, fine – I won't mention it again then, eh?' she snapped, before stomping off.

'Ever!' she added huffily over her shoulder as she swept out of the room, slamming the door behind her.

Dirk stared after her, a confused look on his face.

'Humans!' he muttered under his breath.

There was another knock ont he door. 'What now!' said Dirk, and in came Christopher. He sat on the bed.

'I was outside – I heard everything,' said Chris.

266

'Spying on me now, eh?' said Dirk, watching a green wine gum turn slowly black as it was infused with the Tears of Hag.

'You know you said you loved Sooz, back in that cave?' said Chris.

'Yes,' said Dirk.

'Is it true?' said Chris.

Dirk blinked for a moment, unsure, before saying, 'Of course not!'

Chris frowned. Dirk had hesitated there for just that little bit too long. 'But you cried, when you said it. Your eyes – you know, you really meant it.'

'Oh, that!' said Dirk looking at Chris. 'That was just cave dust.'

'What?' said Chris, half horrified, half relieved.

'Yeah, I rubbed dust into my eyes. Had to make it convincing, right?' said Dirk, with a little mischievous grin on his face.

Chris laughed. 'You little sneaker!' he said.

'Well, yes, indeed,' said Dirk. 'But don't tell Sooz! Not ever, right?'

'OK,' said Chris. 'I won't.'

'How is she, anyway?' said Dirk, returning to his task of spiking wine gums.

'She's fine. Mostly, she's just really, really embarrassed about it all. Being a Vampire and... everything.'

'Why? She made for a great Vampire. Fantastic! And she got us the tears – it all worked out fine in the end,' said Dirk. 'What's there to be embarrassed about?'

'Well...you know, all that love stuff...and...that,' said Chris.

Dirk turned back to Chris again. 'Love stuff? What do you mean?.'

Chris shrugged and looked away.

Dirk turned back to the wine gums. He shook his head. 'Humans! I'll never understand them!

'Well,' continued Dirk, 'they're done, the Wine Gums of Doom are ready. Now I just have to make sure Hasdruban eats some. That psycho bloke, Dr Wings, got him hooked on them apparently, so shouldn't be too hard.'

# The Headmaster's Study...of Death!

The next day, Dirk stood outside the headmaster's study. Mrs Batelakes was with him – it was she who was 'taking him to see the headmaster' because he'd handed in homework that Skinrash the Goblin had done for him. Homework that was rude, disrespectful, gross etc etc, and had earned him this appointment with destiny.

It was the big face-off. Dirk knew what the headmaster had in store for him – a pit trap and a row of wooden stakes. But what Hasdruban didn't know was that Dirk had rewired the trap to backfire. Maybe it would zap Hasdruban long enough so that Dirk could force a wine gum down his throat.

'Well, we shall see who triumphs, won't we?' said Dirk, putting his fingers together in front of his chest. He was about to unleash a 'Mwah, hah, hah!' when he caught Mrs Batelakes glaring at him.

He smiled back at her. She looked away quickly and rapped on the door. It opened almost immediately. The headmaster stood there, dressed in his white suit and hat, long white beard and improbably bushy eyebrows. And dark glasses. With white frames.

'Ah, Dr Hasdruban,' said Mrs Batelakes, 'I've got Dirk Lloyd here for the disciplinary hearing.'

'Right, right,' said Hasdruban. 'I can take it from here, Mrs Batelakes,' he went on breezily. 'You may go!'

'Umm...that's not really...procedure...I should be there,' stuttered Mrs Batelakes.

'Don't trouble yourself! I'll deal with it, really, off you go, Mrs Batelakes,' said Hasdruban.

Mrs Batelakes stuttered. 'But...but...'

'But nothing, Mrs Batelakes! I'm the headmaster here, and I'm telling you, I'll deal with it, all right?' said Hasdruban brusquely, his beard almost quivering with power.

'Yes, headmaster,' said Mrs Batelakes, cowed by his authority. White Wizards were like that. She looked down at Dirk, frowned, and then stepped away.

'Come in...Dirk,' said Hasdruban, stepping aside

and gesturing at the seat in front of his oak desk.

Dirk smiled up at him. 'Hello...headmaster,' he said as he walked in, strode over and sat on the chair he knew to be a trap, confident that it would all blow up in the Wizard's face.

Hasdruban smiled. He shut the door, stepped over to the great throne behind the desk, and sat down.

'Well,' said Hasdruban. 'Here we are.' His hand moved down to hover just below the desktop.

Dirk knew exactly where that hand was – ready to push the button that would tip his chair over and pitch him onto rows of sharpened wooden stakes in the pit below. Or so Hasdruban thought.

'Indeed,' said Dirk. 'Wine gum? he said, putting a bag of them on the desk in front of the headmaster.

Hasdruban looked down at them. 'Hah! You think I would accept a gift from the Evil One so easily? You

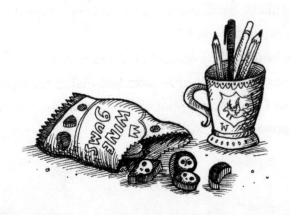

must take me for a fool!' he said.

Dirk shrugged. He hadn't expected that to work, of course, but worth a try. The electric shock ploy was a much better bet, anyway.

'Well, headmaster,' said Dirk, 'I'd like to apologise for the quality of my homework; it was very rude and disrespectful to Mrs Batelakes.'

Dr Hasdruban threw back his head and laughed out loud. 'Priceless, Dark One, priceless! I mean, who cares about Battleaxe, anyway, the dried-up old crone!'

'Now, now,' said Dirk, 'you shouldn't be rude about your teachers, should you, headmaster? She'll have you up before one of those human employment tribunal things if you're not careful!'

'Indeed!' laughed Hasdruban heartily. 'They're mad here, aren't they? All of them, mad as Goblins after too much sugar. Like that one of yours – what was it called? Skinrash or something? I presume it did the work for you?'

Dirk nodded.

'Always one of your weaknesses, your minions. Orcs and Goblins – hopelessly unreliable!' said Hasdruban.

'Maybe. But then again, what about Orcs in tanks? Ever thought about that?' said Dirk.

Hasdruban's eyes narrowed. 'I have indeed. That is why I can't leave you alive here, don't you see?'

'Ah,' said Dirk, finally beginning to understand why Hasdruban was so implacable in his pursuit – fear. Of course, they all feared the Dark Lord and his cunning, his evil genius.

Dirk put his fingers together and smiled. 'It was all so much more straightforward back home, wasn't it?' he said.

'Quite,' nodded Hasdruban. 'Here there's just so much...stuff!'

The White Wizard and the Dark Lord fell silent. They stared at each for a few moments.

'Well,' said Hasdruban, 'It's been nice reminiscing, but I really must get on.'

Dirk nodded. 'Indeed,' he said, 'I understand.'

Hasdruban gestured with his head. Dirk frowned, not understanding. Hasdruban jerked his head again, up at the corner of the room. Dirk looked over. In the top right hand corner he could see something...a little red light blinking.

A CCTV camera! That meant...Hasdruban had

seen everything...seen him creep in, plant the axe, sit in his chair – rewire the pit trap!!! He knew...

'Nooo!' cried Dirk, as Hasdruban hit the button, releasing the trap door. Desperately, Dirk tried to leap aside as the floor fell away beneath him, but it was too late! He began to fall.

Hasdruban crowed with delight.

At the last moment, Dirk was able to catch hold of an arm of the chair that was bolted to the trap door. He was hanging on by the skin of his teeth! He looked down. The wooden stakes were sharp and deadly – he could almost hear them begging him to jump down and say hello, to feel their sharp caress. Dirk clung to the chair. He looked up.

Hasdruban was standing at the edge of the pit, looking down at him. Dirk gulped. He could barely hold on – all Hasdruban had to do was kick him or poke him with the cane a few times, and he'd fall to his doom.

Dirk was defenceless.

Hasdruban clapped his hands together in glee. 'Oh, joy, oh glory! How I've waited for this moment, how perfect it is! They'll remember me as the greatest White Wizard of all time, the one who finally slew the Dark Lord!'

Dirk looked up at him, mind racing. He couldn't think of a way out... This was it. The end. He was going to die after all.

Hasdruban leaned back against the desk, and folded his arms. 'This is almost too much fun,' he said, grinning like an idiot. 'I can't quite bring myself to finish it!'

Dirk's grip began to loosen. He wouldn't be able to hold on much longer.

'You can't blame me for wanting to savour this moment, now can you? Not after all these years!' said Hasdruban.

Without thinking, Hasdruban reached over, picked up a wine gum and popped it into his mouth. He giggled and began to chew.

Suddenly his expression changed. The colour drained from his face. His head twitched, throwing his glasses off, revealing his dark, all-black eyes. He gave an inarticulate cry and put his hands up to his face. Black stuff began to trickle out between his fingers, running down his hands and staining the sleeves of his once immaculate white suit.

Dirk's jaw dropped. He hadn't expected it would

be this radical!

'What's happening to me?' cried the White Wizard, as he fell to his knees, hands and sleeves darkly stained, as if he'd dipped them into a vat of black ink.

Suddenly, Hasdruban's hands fell away, revealing his eyes.

They were bright blue and thoroughly human.

'Oh my! You poor, poor fellow!' he said, as he reached down and pulled Dirk out of the pit. 'There you are, my boy! How are you feeling?'

'Much better, thanks!' said Dirk. His plan had worked – Hasdruban had swallowed the tears, and

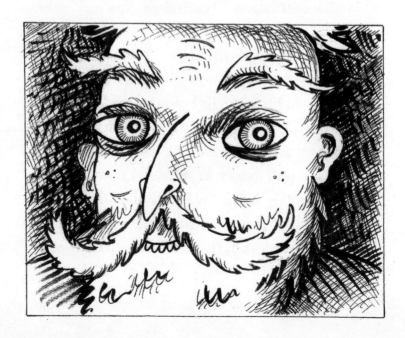

they'd made him feel empathy, care about people, even him!

Dirk put his hands together and laughed.

'Mwah, hah, hah!'

# *Epilogue*

**D**irk sat sprawled across the Throne of Skulls, in the Great Hall of Gloom in the Iron Tower of Despair, beyond the Plains of Desolation, in the Darklands. Except today the Great Hall wasn't really that gloomy at all.

All the lamps had been lit, the statues on either side draped in happy, bright flags and banners, the vaulted ceiling hung with...disco lights. Yes, disco lights, all the way from Earth. Powered by a generator that throbbed and hummed behind the throne.

In the great hall, Goblins, Orcs and humans were dancing to the music of the most famous band in the Darklands – Soozie and the Nightwalkers (actually, currently the only band in the Darklands). They were playing in front of him, on the raised dais of the throne, Sooz on vocals, Gargon on lead guitar, Chris on bass, and Rufino on drums. Agrash had been brought in as well – mostly he used a tambourine. But on one or two songs he came into his own – doing a Goblin rap, or Goblin hip hop, as he called it. And he was pretty good at it too. Called himself Aggy Z.

Dirk was idly stroking the feathers of Dave the Storm Crow, who was perched beside him on the arm of the throne. He was watching the whole show with indulgent amusement. Goblins danced like capering Imps, all elbows and knees, like little green, pot-bellied Morris dancers after drinking way too much coffee. Orcs shifted from foot to foot mostly, or occasionally jumped up and down like electrocuted punk rockers.

Or they'd play air guitar.

Skinrash, dressed in a white waiter's suit, leaned over with a bottle in his hand. 'Top-up of cola, sir?' he said. Dirk waved him away.

It'd been a strange journey, getting here. The tears of the Lady Grieve had worked better than he had expected. Hasdruban had changed completely. He was more like a kindly old man now, filled with wisdom and compassion, rather than an implacable Wizard who would stop at nothing to achieve his goals.

The Light and the Dark had come to terms pretty quickly. Sooz and Dirk had sat down with Hasdruban and the White Witch (she was fine, doing well), and had thrashed out the details. Peace broke out everywhere! Soozville, the town she'd founded when she was Queen of the Darklands was flourishing. Orcs, Goblins, humans and Elves were mostly trading rather than fighting. Sure, there was still trouble and stuff, but no full scale wars. Sooz, Dirk and Chris spent most of their time back on Earth, but they visited the Darklands regularly, at weekends, or in school holidays. They brought useful things to the Darklands and the Commonwealth. Medicine, advanced tools, new ways of growing food. They took back Orc and Goblin arts and crafts to Earth. They sold them to rich people who loved their strangeness, their pagan brutishness and their raw emotion. Also, a popular line in Goth clothing, all put together by Hans the Disembodied Valet[1], as well as a growing line in Moonsilver jewellery.

They'd formed a company, Dark Lord Enterprises, headed up by Rufino. They'd had to train him up a bit, teach him to be a little more like a modern Earth

---

1. See *Dark Lord: A Fiend in Need*. If you haven't read it yet you are a fool, puny human.

person. But not too much – he had a kind of Olde Worlde charm about him that people loved.

Amazingly, Hasdruban had decided to stay on as headmaster of Whiteshields comprehensive. He was turning into a fine headmaster, kind and compassionate, but also firm, with an air of quiet authority. Occasionally he returned to the White Tower, but mostly he wanted to be 'with his children, bless them all. Well, most of them, hah, hah!' as he often said pointedly, looking at Dirk. But only in jest, of course.

Dirk grinned his evil grin, and settled back into his throne, enjoying the music.

Things were going really well...

# Final and Last Epilogue (Honest)

In a lonely bedsit, in a rundown tower block in the cheap side of town, sat the old headmaster, Grousammer, hand on red-raw chin, staring at a bottle on his shelf. The bottle was full of a glistening black liquid he'd found in a puddle in a car park. What was it, and why did he want to drink it?

Slowly, his hand reached for the bottle...

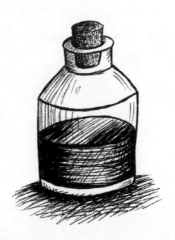

# Acknowledgements

This tome of sheer awesomeness couldn't have been done without...well, ME!

Err...that's it.

The Great Dirk.

# The Author

Originally from a world beyond our own, Dirk Lloyd lives in the town of Whiteshields, in England, where he spends most of his time trying to get out of school and back home to his Iron Tower in the Darklands.

He has been a Dark Lord for more than a thousand years. Some of his achievements include: building the Iron Tower of Despair; raising vast armies of Orcs and Goblins; the waging of great wars; the destruction of many cities; the casting of mighty spells and enchantments; and excelling in English, Science and Maths classes at school.

Now he is a writer. Reviewers who adversely criticise his work may end up joining the others who have not been totally effusive with their praise. Join them in death, that is.

Well, all right, not actual death, but a long

time being tortured in the author's Dungeon of Doom.

Oh, all right, not actually tortured. By the Nine Hells, not even incarceration in my Dungeon of Doom either, OK?

They will be in trouble though. Oh yes, most definitely! They might get cursed, or suffer the Charm of Sudden Baldness or the Cantrip of Uncontrollable Flatulence. Possibly.

So there.

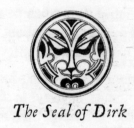

*The Seal of Dirk*

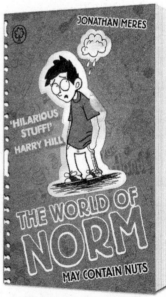